Probiotics

Protection Against Infection

Using Nature's Tiny Warriors
To Stem Infection and Fight Disease

By Casey Adams, Ph.D.

Probiotics—Protection Against Infection:
Using Nature's Tiny Warriors To Stem Infection and Fight Disease
Copyright © 2009 Casey Adams
SACRED EARTH PUBLISHING
Wilmington, Delaware
http://www.sacredearthpublishers.com
All rights reserved.
Printed in USA
Front cover image © Irochka-Fotolia
Back cover "Vitruvian Man" by Leonardo da Vinci, est. 1487
Original illustrations by Virginia Callow

Publishers Cataloging in Publication Data
Adams, Casey
Probiotics—Protection Against Infection:
Using Nature's Tiny Warriors To Stem Infection and Fight Disease

First Edition

1. Medicine. 2. Health.
    Bibliography and References; Index

Library of Congress Control Number: 2009939691

Paperback ISBN-13: 978-0-9816045-5-8
Ebook ISBN-13: 978-1-936251-00-1

*For those who have opened their minds to the
Balance living within nature.*

Table of Contents

Introduction

Every body is infected. How? Simply by eating and breathing. Simply by putting anything into our mouths. With every breath, we breathe in millions of airborne bacteria. With every bite from every fork, we bring in billions of foodborne microbes of different species, shapes and sizes.

What happens to all these infectious microorganisms? Some might be taken out by our immune system. Some might be removed with tooth brushing or mouth washing. The rest are free to invade every body crevice and organ, including the intestines, liver, joints, lungs and urinary tract.

These microorganisms are making us sick. We are finding infections increasing worldwide despite our antibiotics, antimicrobial soaps, mouthwashes, disinfectants, chlorine pools and germophobia.

We are also finding that some of these microorganisms are getting stronger. They are adapting to our antimicrobial ways.

What do we do now?

It is time to fight fire with fire. It is time to unleash nature's sworn enemies of these pathogenic microbes: our friendly microorganisms. It is time to colonize our own microbes against this pathogenic invasion. It is time to put nature back to its original order. Where the strong survive. It is time to employ the evolutionarily stronger probiotic bacteria—who have won the wars and battles against pathogens for thousands of years.

We have excluded the probiotics from our arsenal for too long. In fact, we have unknowingly broken the backs of many of our probiotic colonies. Our antimicrobial lifestyles have knocked probiotics back a step and allowed the pathogens to get stronger.

However, it's not too late. As long as we act now.

This book clarifies not only what probiotics are and do, but how they cooperate with our immune system to combat a multitude of infections and disease pathologies. I have reviewed over 600 *human clinical studies* on probiotics to arrive at the conclusions made in this book.

I have also reviewed hundreds of sometimes-cruel animal studies. For the most part, the conclusions made here do not utilize these animal studies. This is not only done on moral grounds. Research has increasingly found that probiotics act differently within different organisms. Animals house different species and strains from humans with a few exceptions. As we will see, probiotics also render different effects among different people with different diseases, infections or weaknesses.

Probiotics are not simply supplements to take when we have indigestion or nausea. They are complex living creatures that symbiotically inhabit our bodies. They deserve a scientific examination focused upon their unique colonizing activities and complex symbiotic relationships with the human immune system and human disease.

— *Casey Adams (cadams@realnaturalhealth.com)*

Microbes Everywhere

We are surrounded by microorganisms. Trillions upon trillions of bacteria, fungi, viruses, parasites, nanobacteria and extremophiles live within our clothes, cars, bathrooms, beds, floors, air, and all over our bodies. Just about everything we touch has millions of microbes living on it. Bacteria also live in and around just about every food. Our bodies are also densely populated with bacteria. There are more bacteria in our bodies than there are cells.

This situation has not changed for millions of years. Bacteria have been living amongst us and other creatures of our planet through the duration. Not only that, but for most of humankind's existence, we slept on earthen floors and straw beds. We farmed in our bare feet or in sandals made of rope. We crapped in holes in the ground and ate with our fingers. We drank out of the streams with our hands, and used twigs to brush our teeth.

How is it that over the past century we have become so fearful of bacteria? How is it that we now live in disinfectant-cleaned houses, and wash our hands with antibacterial soaps, and we still have a mortal fear of bacteria? How is it that despite these measures, we are still becoming infected?

Today, despite our various antibiotics, antivirals, disinfectants, mouthwashes and antiseptic cleaners, infectious diseases are on the rise. Rates of tuberculosis, influenza, shingles, mononucleosis, cytomegalovirus, malaria, HIV, AIDS and herpes are increasing worldwide. Estimates have calculated that 80% of the U.S. population may be infected with Herpes Simplex 1, while some 45 million are infected with the genital variety, HS2. More than half the world's population harbors *Helicobacter pylori* bacteria. About 1.5 million Americans are infected with sexually transmitted diseases gonorrhea, syphilis or chlamydia. Over 33 million people around the world were theoretically infected with

HIV in 2005—a rise of 16% per year. In the U.S. alone, there are about 40,000 new cases of HIV documented every year. About one third of the world's population is infected with the tuberculosis bacterium. Every year about 6 million people die from TB according to the CDC. Millions more are infected with waterborne diseases throughout the world.

Bacterial Realization

Western medicine had no idea that bacteria even existed until 1673, when Dutch scientist Antony van Leeuwenhoek began writing letters to the Royal Society of London about the images he was seeing in his newly invented microscope. In 1674, Leeuwenhoek wrote about the bacteria he found on a nearby lake. He said they were "wound serpent-wise and orderly arranged, after the manner of the copper or tin worms." In 1683, Leeuwenhoek described bacteria found from the plaque between his teeth. He described "many very little living animalcules."

Research on bacteria continued in a curious manner until several scientists like Edward Jenner, Ignaz Semmelweis, Friedrich Henle and Louis Pasteur proposed that disease was caused primarily by microorganisms.

The germ-disease relationship was not a new one, however. Even before Leeuwenhoek saw his 'animalcules,' ancient physicians had proposed that many diseases were caused by tiny organisms. Some ancient medicines contemplated invading disease forces, and some even employed vaccination techniques. The prominent middle eastern physician Avicenna discussed infectious disease in his 1020 A.D. *Canon of Medicine.* Italian physician Fracastorius proposed that syphilis and typhus were the result of contagious germs. Thousands of years earlier, Ayurvedic medicine pinpointed the existence of infective cells among disease pathologies.

Western medical science realized the connection between the immune system and these infective cells in 1796, when Dr. Edward Jenner scraped smallpox blisters from an infected worker who contracted the cowpox from milking cows. The pus was collected onto some wood and injected into the arms of an eight-year old boy. Twenty-three others were injected after the boy survived. The reduction of smallpox incidence among the injected group was noticeable, and the modern-day technique of vaccination was born.

Types of Microbes

Fungi	Yeasts, molds and others; over 100,000 species; live in earth, air, water and damp, moist environments; can infect the body via food, water, air, and skin
Bacteria	Single-celled organisms; live in water, earth, air, on and inside other living organisms; can infect via food, water, air, and skin
Viruses	Non-living; genetic mutation triggers; exist in water, earth, air and skin; infect by altering cellular DNA, and spreading through ongoing cell division and mutation
Mycoplasmas	Ancient slow-moving bacteria; live primarily on earth and water; infect mostly via food, water and touch
Parasites	Tiny organisms that infect and live within another living organism. Includes worms, protozoa and amoeba
Thermophiles	Opportunistic bacteria that can live in very hot environments, such as deserts, boiling water or even in ovens
Psychophiles	Opportunistic bacteria that can live in the very cold, such as the artic or in freezers
Nanobacteria	Extremely small bacteria that typically have a hard calcium shell. Are thought to cause some diseases considered autoimmune.

Today we are dealing with a multitude of infections from all of these types of microorganisms. Growing infectious diseases from this list include lyme disease (*Borrelia burgdorferi*), pneumonia, staphylococcus, streptococcus, salmonella, *E. coli*, cholera, listeria, salmonella, shigellia, dengue fever, yellow fever, tuberculosis, cryptosporidiosis, hepatitis, rabies and others. Many of these microorganisms are growing despite our antibiotic and antiviral medications. Some are growing because of unsafe sex, unclean water or changes in land use. Many are growing because of new opportunities arising from our destruction of nature. Many are becoming resistent to our antibiotics. These are often referred to as *superbugs.*

One of the more dangerous of these superbugs is methicillin-resistant *Staphylococcus aureus* (MRSA). MRSA rates are on the rise, and nearly every hospital—the crown jewels of our antimicrobial kingdom—is infected with MRSA. In a 2007 survey of 1200 U.S. hospitals, 46 of every 1,000 hospital inpatients are colonized or infected with MRSA, with 75% of those being infected. Among the general population, the incidence of MRSA has skyrocketed from 24 cases per 100,000 people in 2000 to 164 cases per 100,000 people in 2005 (Hota *et al.* 2007). This means that MRSA is infecting nearly seven times the number of people it did in 2000.

The virulence of *Staphylococcus aureus* was first realized in 1929 by Alexander Fleming, a microbiologist who cultured a combination of *Staphylococcus aureus* in the vicinity of a growing mold. He noticed that the penicillin mold would kill some bacteria and not others. Fleming soon realized that *Staphylococcus aureus* adapted quickly to the penicillin. It became resistant. Even to this day, *Staphylococcus aureus* is still one of the most antibiotic-resistant bacteria.

Staphylococcus aureus is also one of the most lethal bacteria known to man. It secretes three cell-killing toxins: alpha toxin, beta toxin and leukocidin. Together these poisons bind to and dissolve cell membranes, allowing cytoplasm and cell contents to leak out. This, of course, immediately kills the cell. The immune system also has difficulty attacking and removing *Staphylococcus aureus* because it secretes enzymes that neutralize the immune system's attack strategies. *Staphylococcus aureus* adapts very quickly, so the more we throw at it, the stronger it becomes.

Infectious bacteria are not always suspected—or even detected—in many diseases. Increasingly, we are finding that many common diseases are caused or worsened by bacteria or fungal infections. We are also seeing an increase in many degenerative diseases connected to infection—including cardiovascular disease, arthritis, ulcer, irritable bowel syndrome, asthma, allergies and chronic fatigue syndrome.

A few diseases linked to microorganisms:

Disease	Some Suspected Microbes
Stroke and cardiovascular diseases	*Helicobacter. pylori* *Treponema pallidum* (syphilis) *Staphylococcus aureus* *Enterococci faecalis* *Streptococcus* spp. Herpes Simplex (I and II) *Pneumonococcal aerogenes* *Candida albicans* *Streptococcus mutans* *Escherichia coli* *Chlamydia pneumonia* *Porphyromonas gingivalis* *Tannerella forsynthensis* *Prevotella intermedia*
Gallstones	Eubacteria *Clostridium* spp.
Ulcers, ulcerative colitis and Crohn's	*Helicobacter pylori* *Clostridium* spp. *E. coli* *Mycobacterium pneumoniae*

Cancers	*Staphylococcus aureus*
	Enterococci faecalis
	Streptococcus spp.
	Pneumonococcal aerogenes
	Streptococcus mutans
	E. coli
	mammary tumor virus
	papilloma virus (HPV)
	H. pylori
	Heptitis B
Diabetes	Coxackle B virus
	Cytomegalovirus
	Salmonella osteomyelitis
	others suspected (see arthritis below)
Arthritis	*Bacteroides fragilis*
	Borrelia burgdorferi
	Brucella melitensis
	Brucellae spp.
	Campylobacter jejuni
	Chlamydia trachomatis
	Clostridium difficile
	Corynebacterium striatum
	Cryptococcal pyarthrosis
	Gardnerella vaginalis
	Kingella kingae
	Listeria monocytogenes
	Moraxella canis
	Mycobacterium lepromatosis
	Mycobacterium marinum
	Mycobacterium terrae
	Mycoplasma arthritidis
	Mycoplasma hominis
	Mycoplasma leachii sp.
	Neisseria gonorrhoeae
	Ochrobactrum anthropi
	Pasteurella multocida

	Pneumocystis jiroveci
	Porphyromonas gingivalis
	Prevotella bivia
	Prevotella intermedia
	Prevotella loescheii
	Pseudomonas aeruginosa
	Pyoderma gangrenosum
	Roseomonas gilardii
	Salmonella entertidis
	Scedosporium prolificans
	Serratia fonticola
	Sphingomonas paucimobilis
	Staphylococcus aureus
	Staphylococcus lugdunensis
	Streptococcus agalactiae
	Streptococcus equisimilis
	Streptococcus pneumoniae
	Streptococcus pyogenes
	Streptococcus uberis
	Tannerella forsynthensis
	Treponema pallidum
	Vibrio vulnificus
	Yersinia enterocolitica
Alzheimer's	*Chlamydia pneumoniae*
	Borna virus
	H. pylori
	Spirochetes
	Herpes simplex I
	picornavirus

Overgrowths of yeasts like *Candida albicans* can also contribute to or be a primary cause for a number of diseases. Research has found that in some cases, *Candida albicans* can grow conjunctively with *Staphylococcus aureus*, resulting in the accelerated growth of both. This can result in a variety of diseases caused by combined yeast and bacteria infections. Viruses and bacteria can also grow in combination. We see this in many of the fatalities from the swine flu and other influenzas. Deaths often occur in immunosuppressed patients with concurrent bacteria infections.

Teeth and Gum Bacteria

Multiple pathogenic microorganisms can grow and prosper within the mouth, teeth and gums. These include *Streptococcus mutans, Streptococcus pyogenes, Porphyromonas gingivalis, Tannerella forsynthensis* and *Prevotella.* Additional microbes can grow within root canals. Root canals provide protected spaces for bacterial growth. Bacteria infecting root canals can include a variety of steptococci, staphylococci, and even dangerous spirochetes such as *Borrelia burgdorferi* among many others. Just about any bacteria that can infect the body internally can hibernate inside root canals. Because root canals are enclosed and the tissues around them die, the immune system cannot reach these areas to remove bacteria. As a result, a growing number of diseases are now being associated with root canal-harbored bacteria.

As these microbial populations grow, they not only can infect teeth and gums with gingivitis: They can also infect various other parts of the body. Infected gums have been implicated in a variety of fatal disorders, including heart disease, lung disease, liver disease, kidney disease, septic arthritis and others. A recent report from the Jos University Teaching Hospital in Nigeria (Adoga *et al.* 2009) reported that, "Most often the cause of cervical necrotizing fascitis is of dental origin." Necrotizing fascitis is a growing lethal infection of multiple bacteria that rapidly destroy tissues around the body, causing death very quickly.

The Anti-Microbial Society

This seemingly unbridled growth in microorganisms and infectious diseases continues despite the fact that our use of prescriptive and over the counter antibiotics, antifungals, antivirals, antiseptic soaps, and cleaning disinfectants has dramatically increased over the past few decades.

Today children receive more than thirty vaccinations for practically every type of infection with a history of risk to children. Adult vaccines are also on the increase. Today's vaccine lineups include polio, measles, mumps, rubella, chickenpox, rotavirus, tetanus, pertussis, meningitis, diphtheria, hepatitis A and B, influenza, and now the human papillomavirus vaccine.

Most agree that vaccinations have reduced the incidence levels of many debilitating and fatal infections. Today, however, there is a critical backlash from a growing segment of American families. Many parents have begun to oppose the number and frequency of these vaccinations. There are also several childhood conditions that are now being thought to relate to the ingredients, quality, content and/or frequency of vaccinations now being given to children. These suspected conditions include allergies, autism and attention deficit syndrome. Conventional medicine largely disputes this theory. Parents and reduced-vaccination advocates point to the dramatic increase of autism over the past two decades—from one out of thousands to one out of hundreds of children.

While this debate rages on, there is no argument that microbial diseases garner significant attention from both government authorities and parents. Microbes are considered enemy number one by the Centers for Disease Control and government anti-terrorism officials. This concern for outbreaks and pandemics has put microbial diseases on the front pages of many newspapers and news broadcasts.

At the same time, the use of antibiotics has soared over the past few decades. Today, over 3,000,000 pounds of pure antibiotics are taken by humans annually in the United States. This is complemented by the approximately 25,000,000 pounds of antibiotics given to animals each year.

Meanwhile, many of these antibiotics either are given in vain or are ineffectual. The Centers for Disease Control states that, *"Almost half of patients with upper respiratory tract infections in the*

U.S. still receive antibiotics from their doctor." This said, the CDC also warns that *"90% of upper respiratory infections, including children's ear infections, are viral, and antibiotics don't treat viral infection. More than 40% of about 50 million prescriptions for antibiotics each year in physicians' offices were inappropriate."*

Indeed, the growing use of antibiotics has also created a Pandora's box of *superbugs*. As bacteria are repeatedly hit with the same antibiotic, they learn to adapt. Just as any living organism does (yes, bacteria are alive), bacteria learn to counter and resist repeatedly utilized antibiotics. As a result, many bacteria today are resistant to a variety of antibiotics. This is because bacteria tend to adjust to their surroundings. If they are attacked enough times with a certain challenge, they are likely to figure out how to avoid it and thrive despite it.

This has been the case for a number of other new antibiotic-resistant strains of bacteria. They have simply evolved to become stronger and more able to counteract these antibiotic measures.

This phenomenon has created *multi-drug resistant organisms.* Some of the more dangerous MDROs include species of *Enterococcus, Staphylococcus, Salmonella, Campylobacter, Escherichia coli,* and others. Superbugs such as MRSA are only the tip of the bacterial iceberg.

Another growing infectious bacterium is *Clostridium difficile.* This bacterium will infect the intestines of people of any age. Among children, this is one of the world's biggest killers—causing acute, watery diarrhea. It is also a growing infection among adults. Every year *C. difficile* infects tens of thousands of people in the U.S. according to the Mayo Clinic. Worse, *C. difficile* are increasingly becoming resistant to antibiotics and infections from clostridia are growing in incidence each year.

Summary of Common Antibiotics

Type	Examples	Use and Side Effects
Penicillins	Amoxicillin Ampicillin	*Stapholococcus* spp., *Streptococcus* spp., STDs, *E. coli,*

	Azlocillin	lyme disease, others
	Carbenicillin	*Adverse side effects include skin*
	Cloxacillin	*rashes, allergic reactions and*
	Dicloxacillin	*anaphylactic response, liver dam-*
	Flucloxacillin	*age, kidney damage, brain dam-*
	Mexlocillin	*age, and probiotic die-off*
	Meticillin	
	Nafcillin	
	Oxacillin	
	Penicillin	
	Piperacillin	
Macrolides	Azithromycin	Pneumonia, *Streptococcus* spp.,
	Clarithromycin	mycoplasma infection, Lyme
	Dirithromycin	and others.
	Erythromycin	*Adverse side effects include jaun-*
	Roxithromycin	*dice, liver damage, diarrhea,*
	Troleandomycin	*vomiting, nausea, skin rashes*
	Telithromycin	*and probiotic die-off*
	Spectinomycin	
Aminoglycosides	Amikacin	Gram-negative bacteri, in-
	Gentamicin	cluding *E. coli*, *Klebsiella* and
	Kanamycin	*Pseudomonas.*
	Neomycin	*Adverse side effects include skin*
	Netilmicin	*rashes, kidney damage, hearing*
	Streptomycin	*loss, vertigo, and knocking out*
	Tobramycin	*body's probiotic system*
	Paromomycin	
Glycopeptides	Teicoplanin	Gram-positive bacteria
	Vancomycin	*Side effects similar to above*
Polypeptides	Bacitracin	Gram-positive bacteria
	Colistin	Topical agent or inhaled.
	Polymyxin	*Allergies and probiotic die-off*
Carbapenems	Ertapenem	Broad spectrum (gram-
	Cilastatin	positive and gram-negative)
	Doripenem	*Adverse side effects include*
	Imipenem	*seizures, headaches, rash, aller-*
	Meropenem	*gies, nausea and probiotic die-off*

Quinolones	Ciprofloxacin Enoxacin Gatifloxacin Levofloxacin Moxifloxacin Norfloxacin Ofloxacin	Pneumonia, UTIs, myco- plamas, STDs, others *Adverse side effects include* *peripheral neuropathy, tendon* *rupture, liver damage, nerve* *damage and depleting probiotic* *colonies.*
Tetracyclines	Demeclocycline Doxycycline Minocycline Monocycline Oxytetracycline Tetracycline	STDs, mycoplasmas, acne, malaria, Lyme disease, others *Adverse effects include long-term* *GI damage, liver damage, growth* *stunting, teeth staining, fetal* *toxicity, probiotic die-off.*
Sulfonamides	Co-trimoxazole Mafenide Sulfacetamide Sulfadiazine Sulfamethizole Sulfasalazine Trimethoprim Sulfamethoxazole	Burns, UTIs, dermatitis, acne, fungi, others *Adverse side effects include kid-* *ney failure, decreased white cell* *count, kidney crystals, skin* *rashes, nausea, diarrhea, and* *knocking out probiotic system.*
Cephalosporins	Cefadroxil Cefazolin Cefalexin Cefaclor Cefproxil Cefoxitin Cefdinir Cefditoren Cefotxaxime Cefepime Ceftobiprole	Broad spectrum *Adverse side effects include skin* *rashes, nausea, seizures, head-* *aches, diarrhea, and eliminating* *probiotic colonies.*
Chloamphenicol	Chloamphenicol	Broad spectrum *Averse side effects include ane-* *mia and probiotic die-off*
Clindamycin	Clindamycin	Broad spectrum; acne, *Clostridium, Pseudomonas,* etc.

		Adverse side effects include diarrhea, colitis, vomiting, cramps, rash, itch, contact dermatitis and probiotic die-off
Lincomycin	Lincomycin	Similar to Clindamycin
Ethambutol	Ethambutol	Tuberculosis and others; *Adverse effects: nerve damage, color blindness, probiotic die-off*
Metronidazole	Metronidazole	Giardia, vaginosis; gingivitis; *Adverse effects: nausea, stomatitis, leucopenia, black hair tongue, nerve and probiotic die-off*
Rifampicin	Rafampicin	Gram-positive; mycobacteria *Adverse effects include rash and tear coloring, probiotic die-off*

The reason there are so many antibiotics now is the same reason that many pathogens are becoming resistant to many of our antibiotics: They are *static* strategies in a *living* system. Living systems are adaptive. They *learn* to work around whatever is thrown at them. Meanwhile, each antibiotic we have developed deters microorganisms with the same strategy every time. Some will interfere with the microorganism's cell wall. Others will interfere with the RNA within the cell—at least until they adapt.

How Bacteria Become Antibiotic Resistant

With time, a microorganism can learn to adapt to practically any threat to its survival. In order to protect itself and its colony, a microorganism will gradually learn how to evade the threat. Over many generations, these strategies are passed on and perfected by successive generations.

To illustrate how bacteria become resistant, let's say that that a burglar broke into a house while the family was home. The man of the house grabs a baseball bat and clubs the burglar on the head, and the burglar runs off. A month later, the burglar breaks into the same house again. What do you think the burglar will be wearing this time? A helmet of course!

We should understand that bacteria—even pathogenic bacteria—are living organisms that simply want to survive. Therefore, when they see a mass threat such as an antibiotic, over several generations they will figure out how to work around that antibiotic. They do this through the development of subtle and successive variations to their genes.

We might wonder how bacteria spread their antibiotic resistance. The interesting thing is that bacteria don't only create a genetic variation: They also create a small suitcase-like package of genetic make-over matter called a *plasmid*, with which they can pass on their genetic variation to other bacteria.

The plasmid is often called a *replicon*, because it can be transferred to another bacterium, who will automatically assimilate it into its genetic information. This allows the new bacterium to perfectly replicate the strategies of the source bacterium. Once inside the new bacterium, the plasmid allows the bacterium to perform the workaround to the antibiotic, and be able to pass the plasmid on to yet another bacterium.

Our broad-spectrum antibiotics might be compared to the baseball bat in the analogy above. Once used, bacteria may adapt to that static (antibiotic) tool. Any number of different species can figure out a way around the antibiotic. Once learned, that trick is passed on to other species of bacteria, and soon the antibiotic will be useless against many different species. This ability to learn on an inter-species level provides one of the scariest features about bacteria infections: The ability for different species to grow beyond our ability to control entire legions of many species of cooperative fungi and bacteria.

This also means that antibiotic resistance is not the same in all geographical regions. Plasmid transfer requires direct contact between bacteria. This was illustrated in a 2007 study on antibiotic resistance among several pathogenic bacteria. Gram-positive bacteria isolates were collected from 76 medical centers among nine regions across the U.S. The results indicated that vancomycin resistance in *Enterococcus faecium* ranged from 45.5% in New England to 85.3% in the East South Central U.S. Methicillin-resistant *Staphylococcus aureus* (MRSA) varied from 27.4% in New England to 62.4% in East South Central. Penicillin-resistant *Streptococcus pneumoniae* ranged from 23.3% in the Pacific region to 54.5% in the East South Central region (Denys *et al.* 2007).

This also means that as bacteria continue to travel on animals, humans, trains, buses, and airplanes, they will continue to exchange their learned resistance to our antibiotics. This will inevitably lead to most of our antibiotics becoming useless.

Probiotics provide the solution to this conundrum. How so? Probiotics are also smart living organisms. They are also the sworn enemies to these pathogenic species. In fact, the probiotics and the pathogenic bacteria have been battling it out for billions of years, and the probiotics have been winning! This is evidenced, of course, by the fact that the human race is still alive. This means that probiotics have figured out how to identify each new plasmid, and respond by developing their own strategies and plasmids to combat pathogenic bacteria.

In our burglary analogy, when the burglar comes back in his helmet, the man of the house pulls out another weapon to scare off the burglar. If he comes back again prepared for that weapon, the man devises a new one. This is what living organisms do as they protect their territories. As pathogenic and probiotic bacteria battle it out, they are both creating new strategies to resist each other. As one develops a new strategy, the other will develop yet another one. They both throw their naturally developed antibiotics at each other, and they each respond in kind.

Research has confirmed that probiotics have the same sorts of tools at their disposal. Probiotics can also develop antibiotic resistance just as pathogenic bacteria like MRSA can. Researchers from Sweden's University of Agricultural Sciences (Rosander *et al.* 2008) found that not only could the *Lactobacillus reuteri* probiotic strain easily develop antibiotic resistance: *L. reuteri* also developed plasmids. In their study, they observed *L. reuteri* carrying *two* plasmids that created and passed on antibiotic resistance to tetracycline and lincosamide.

Foodborne Microbes

It seems like once every few months, panic seems to grip the United States population with a new foodborne illness outbreak. The past year witnessed a number of big U.S. recalls and in recent years a variety of foods and beverages were pulled from shelves and restaurants after reports of sicknesses from foodborne bacteria and viruses.

The peanut butter contamination early in 2009 was the largest food recall in U.S. history. After *Salmonella* sickened a few hundred people, billions of dollars of foods—contaminated or not—with even trace amounts of peanut butter, were tossed out. Nine people were thought to have died from complications due to salmonella, and over 20,000 people were thought to have been struck with salmonellosis poisoning. The scare caused many people to entirely give up eating a healthy food. Sales of all types of peanut butters and products with peanuts plunged.

During the summer of 2008, some salsa products were found to contain *Salmonella* after they sickened a few dozen people. In all, there were about 200 hospitalizations, and two deaths. The outbreak forced a huge tomato recall that dearly cost the tomato industry. It was later found that serrano peppers from Mexico were responsible.

In 2007, a *Listeria* outbreak was blamed on milk products coming from a Massachusetts dairy. Two were said to have died from the contamination.

A year later, 8,000 cartons of spinach was recalled from product after a few tested positive for *Salmonella*, even though no illnesses were reported.

In 2006, an outbreak of *E. coli* poisoning was blamed on spinach supplied by a California spinach grower. It was reported that three people might have died from the poisoning, and about 200 persons over two dozen states reported being sickened.

In 1999, *Salmonella* was also found in unpastuerized orange juice from Mexico.

In one of the more sensational *E. coli* outbreaks, apple juice sickened sixty children with one death in the mid-1990s.

Other notable outbreaks of *E. coli* in the past few decades or so have included cookie dough, lettuce, and a variety of meat products like beef. *E coli* infections have also come from drinking water. At the 1998 Washington County, New York Fair, over a thousand people were said to have been sickened, and two people apparently died from drinking the local water.

It is more sensational when a healthy food causes a foodborne outbreak. The majority of outbreaks are meat-related, but these are no longer sensational news. Infectious outbreaks among meats or meat-containing products such as pot-pies, hamburgers, chicken, beef and many other meat products have infected people on a widespread basis over the past decade. *E. coli* O157:H7 in beef alone sickens tens of thousands per year according to the CDC. Sixteen outbreaks in the past three years have been traced back to this pathogen in ground beef. During the summer of 2009 alone, 3,000 grocery stores in 41 states were subject to recalls of contaminated ground beef. *Salmonella* outbreaks have included chicken, scallions, and beef. Testing has also shown that 1 out of 20,000 commercial eggs are contaminated by *Salmonella enteritidis.*

Other bacteria also infect meat products. A *Listeria* outbreak infected thousands from chickens in 2002. Canned fish infected thousands people with botulism in 1992. *Giardia, Shigella, Staphylococcus aureus, Mycobacterium tuberculosis, Yersinia enterocolitica, Campylobacter jejuni, Cryptosporidia* and *Listeria monocytogenes* can also infect food, especially if they are prepared from infected water sources or from infected food handler hands. Some viruses can also infect food. *Calcivirus* or *Norwalk-like virus* infections have been documented, mostly from fish and oysters, but can also be spread through hand contact. *Trichinosis,* quite common in pork, can also seriously sicken.

Ground beef is particularly vulnerable to contamination because most ground beef is made up of meat from different slaughterhouses in different locations, including outside the country. One study showed that commercially sold ground beef patties were a conglomeration of trimmings and scraps from slaughterhouses and processors from Nebraska, Texas, Uruguay, South Dakota and Wisconsin.

Few of these meat grinders are required to test for foodborne pathogens like *E. coli* and *Salmonella.* A study published in the *New York Times* found that many of the larger slaughterhouses even try to sell only to those processors that agree not to test their incoming meat for *E. coli,* for fear of setting off a large recall. Meanwhile, the USDA and FDA do little or no direct testing, relying instead upon the manufacturers to test their own products. Food safety expert and University of Minnesota professor Dr. Jeffrey Bender commented, saying that, "Ground beef is not a completely safe product." (Moss 2009)

These are but a few of the many recalls and outbreaks of foodborne bacteria over recent years in the U.S.

What is going on here? Should we shudder when we buy and eat commercially prepared foods? Should we trust the inspection, pasteurization and sterilization processes supposedly supervised by the FDA and state health departments? In other words, can we trust our foods, and if so, which ones?

There are many reasons connected to infection occurrence, outside of the contamination issue. One reason is that there is more mass distribution of food from one location to many locations throughout the U.S. This magnifies the potential for infection. Most food now travels well beyond outside of its current area of production.

Our ancestors were limited in their exposure simply because they were more in contact with their food. Their food was also fresher. Now not only do manufacturers have to guarantee a food is safe after packaging, but they have to guarantee it through a lengthy journey through various distributors and warehouses, any one of which could contaminate or otherwise mishandle the product. This has forced manufacturers to come closer and closer to sterilizing our foods—and spoiling their nutrient levels—for fear of contamination.

Food contamination can come from many sources. The harvesting and plant environment, the cleanliness of workers, food washing techniques and water quality can all infect food. Even a sanitary facility can give rise to many microbes, and these can get into the food during preparation. In the case of the peanut outbreak, the walls and ceiling tiles of the peanut factory were found to be moldy. Microbes can also reside within filling systems and packaging equipment, and within packaging materials.

As we compare the statistics between different countries and foodborne illness outbreaks in other countries, we find a trend. Americans had 26,000 cases of foodborne illness for every 100,000 persons in the U.S. between 1996 and 1998. The UK had 3,400 cases per 100,000 people. France had 1,210 cases per 100,000 people. Why are Americans having more foodborne illnesses than the UK or France?

Let's look at this further. In the U.S., 111 per 100,000 people were hospitalized for foodborne illness. In France, 24 per 100,000 were hospitalized. In the U.S., 1.7 people died per 100,000 people from foodborne illness during that period. In France, .9 per 100,000 people died from foodborne illness.

The first question of why there are more cases in the U.S. per unit of population is overshadowed by why there are also so many more deaths and hospitalizations for foodborne illness in the U.S.? What is about the United States that gets more people sick from their food? Perhaps it is not in the food at all.

The Invasion

So many different species of microbes can reside within our foods. *Clostrium botulinum* can grow in food or juice containers, especially cans, to produce a sometimes-deadly disease called botulism. *Campylobacter* species is one of the most common foodborne bacteria, usually prevalent in meat. This causes diarrhea, fever and cramping, but rarely death. The *E. coli* O157:H7 bacteria can sometimes be lethal (verocytosis) in immune-suppressed people, but for most people it causes a little nausea and a few days of diarrhea. *Salmonella* is prevalent in the intestines of many wildlife, including birds, reptiles and other animals (including humans). It too will mostly cause a little nausea and diarrhea in an otherwise healthy person.

While warm, moist environments are favored, bacteria can survive extreme environments. They can survive in the fridge, the freezer and even in low-oxygen vacuum containers. In colder temperatures, bacteria can incubate. A little warm moisture will revive billions of bacteria into colony formation. Many foodborne bacteria colonize via the release of spores, which can survive even the harshest conditions—including pasteurization. A single spore can quickly grow into an entire colony of bacteria.

Microbial Food Fight

Today we think we are evading bacteria with our arsenal of antimicrobial barriers. We think that our chlorination, antibacterial soaps and disinfected floors will keep these invasions away.

Most of us have a false sense of security in our manufactured foods. We think that because most manufacturers pasteurize our food, they will be bacteria-free. This is far from reality.

French chemist Louis Pasteur developed pasteurization in the 1860s to disprove the notion of spontaneous generation—a theory that some put forth to explain how life arose from chemicals. Pasteurization is by far the process that commercial food manufacturers use the most to reduce bacteria in foods and beverages. Most, but certainly not all bacteria colonies are removed with this process.

Today pasteurization is used for practically every commercially packaged food that has significant water or moisture content. This includes practically every shelf-stable canned food, sauce and mix in jars. Today even vegetables, nuts, fruit, prepackaged dinners, entrees, and refrigerated juices are also commonly pasteurized.

Pasteurization is the treatment of a food to the point where a large percentage of the bacteria are eliminated. There are five basic types of pasteurization: *Holder* or *steam* pasteurization, *high temperature* or *flash* pasteurization, *ultra high* pasteurization, *irradiation* pasteurization, and *gas* pasteurization.

Holder, vat, tunnel or steam pasteurization requires bringing the food or liquid to 140-145 degrees Fahrenheit for a period of about thirty minutes. For many foods, this takes place by heating the product after being packaged. Cans, for example, will be heated in an airtight, jacketed chamber. This might follow additional kettle cooking and "hot-filling."

Steam or tunnel pasteurization is used for many sauces and juices, especially those packaged in glass. Before this stage the product may still be heated and hot-packed. Following filling, the jar or container is sealed and placed on a conveyor belt, which carries it through a heated tunnel. The tunnel bakes the product while hot water is sprayed onto the package. This creates a blanket of hot steam in the tunnel, heating the package and its contents to the desired temperature. Following the hot steam, a cooling section of the tunnel sprays colder water on it to cool the product down.

Flash or high pasteurization (also called HTST for "high temperature, short time") is done primarily on liquids or slurry products. HTST will take the liquid to 160-165 degrees for 15 seconds. For some liquids, the temperature and time is different. Regular milk (non-UHT), for example, is typically pasteurized by heating to 120 degrees for about 20 seconds. HTST is typically done by running the product through a series of pipes and heat exchanger plates that boost its temperature quickly. Following this, the product is filled into the container. Some processors will still run it through another heating tunnel after packing to prevent contamination in the package. Note that the term "flash pasteurized" has been used in marketing to imply a system somehow less damaging than high temp pasteurization.

Ultra pasteurization (UP) will heat the liquid higher, sometimes over 200 degrees F, for a few seconds. Time and temperature can range, depending upon the product and the desired outcome. The intense heat of ultra pasteurization typically doubles the shelf life compared to regular pasteurization.

Then there is ultra high temperature pasteurization, or UHT. UHT will usually heat the food or liquid to about 280 degrees F, but only for a period from a half-second to two or three seconds. This is done mostly for liquids, which are run through a number of extreme heat exchanging chambers before being packaged — usually in an 'aseptic' vacuum package. UHT will typically allow a product to be put on the dry shelf for an extended period. This process is also sometimes incorrectly referred to as sterilization.

Irradiation pasteurization is a growing method of reducing microorganisms from produce and other products. Because it does not raise the temperature of the product as high as other methods, it is also sometimes marketed as "cold pasteurization." Imported produce is now commonly irradiated as shipments arrive by air or by sea. Increasingly, large U.S. food producers irradiate their raw products because the appearance and flavor of the product is often better preserved. The most common method uses cobalt-60 radiation. X-rays and gamma radiation are also used. Irradiation is not allowed in organic produce. Worker health in irradiation plants has also been a concern.

Gas pasteurization is used for a limited number of foods. Almonds and other nuts, for example are sometimes pasteurized by gassing them with either propylene oxide or hot steam. Organic nut production, of course, does not allow propylene oxide.

For milk and other liquids, UHT and HTST also accompany homogenization. Homogenization blends and mixes the product significantly, which can alter molecular polarity and structure.

Commercial foods that have higher acidity (usually with a pH of less than 4.6) and/or intense sugar content may be able to skip pasteurization. Commercial manufacturers usually have to pass a state pH test before they can package a liquid product without pasteurization. Most acidic juices like orange, apple, carrot and berry used to be commercially available fresh. After the '90s apple juice outbreak, many regulators began requiring HTST for mass-distributed refrigerated fruit juices. Raw milk has been readily available commercially for thousands of years until recently. Before government regulators have increasingly banned or restricted commercial distribution of raw packaged foods, raw milk was a wonderfully natural, probiotic beverage.

A few foods that are commercially unpasteurized include some balsamic vinegar, kombucha tea, hummus, honey, maple syrup, and a variety of probiotic-fermented foods. We might ask why fermented and probiotic foods can escape pasteurization? Because they've been naturally acidified by probiotic bacteria to a degree that discourages growth of foodborne microbes. As we will discuss, probiotics consume sugars and carbohydrates, and secrete healthy acids, which also repel pathogenic organisms.

Pasteurization, on the other hand, does not by any means kill all the microbes present. It can significantly reduce it, yes. At best, pasteurization systems will lower *plate count* levels down by about 99%. This means, for example, if there are 1 trillion bacteria colony-forming units in the food in the beginning, there might still be 10 billion CFU left after pasteurization. For HST pasteurization, the removal rate is higher, about 99.9% removal.

This means for a 1 trillion CFU initial population, there would be a billion CFU population left after heat treatment.

Now we might ask; how many colony-forming units would it take of a bacteria species to make us sick? A billion is plenty, as long as there is food in the form of sugars and carbohydrates, and a reasonable growth temperature.

Is Pasteurized Food Healthy?

This is an important question. Most nutrients are heat-sensitive. Vitamin C, fat-soluble vitamins A, E and B vitamins and even certain amino acids are depleted during pasteurization. Important plant nutrients such as anthocyanins and polyphenols are also reduced during pasteurization, along with various enzymes. Proteins are denatured or broken down when heated for long. While this can aid in amino acid absorption, it can also form unrecognized peptide combinations. In milk, for example, nutritious whey protein, or lactabumin, will denature into various peptide combinations, some of which are not readily absorbed.

A 2008 study on strawberry puree from the University of Applied Sciences in Switzerland showed a 37% reduction in vitamin C and a significant loss in antioxidant potency after pasteurization. A 1998 study from Brazil's Universidade Estadual de Maringa determined that Barbados cherries lost about 14% of their vitamin C content after pasteurization. During heat treatment, vitamin C will also convert to dehydroascorbic acid together with a loss of bioflavonoids.

A 2008 study at Spain's Cardenal Herrera University determined that glutathione peroxidase—an important antioxidant contained in milk—was significantly reduced by pasteurization. In 2006, this university also released a study showing that lysine content was significantly decreased by milk pasteurization. A 2005 study at the Universidade Federal do Rio Grande determined that pasteurizing milk reduced vitamin A (retinol) content from an average of 55 micrograms to an average of 36.6 micrograms. A study at North Carolina State University in 2003 determined that HTST pasteurization significantly reduced conjugated linoleic acid (CLA) content—an important fatty acid in milk shown to reduce cancer and encourage good fat metabolism.

A 2006 study on bayberries at the Southern Yangtze University determined that plant antioxidants such as anthocyanins and polyphenolics were reduced from 12-32% following UHT pasteurization. Polyphenols are the primary nutrients in fruits and vegetables that render anticarcinogenic and antioxidant effects.

Probably the most important loss from pasteurization is enzyme content. Diary and plant foods contain a variety of enzymes that aid in the assimilation or catalyzing of nutrients and antioxidants. These include xanthenes, lysozymes, lipases, oxidases, amylases, lactoferrins and many others. Food enzymes also deter the formation of certain microbes, and help keep product from spoiling. The body uses food enzymes in various ways. Some enzymes, such as papain from papaya and bromelain from pineapples, dissolve artery plaque and reduce inflammation. While the body makes many of its own enzymes, it also absorbs some food enzymes or uses their components to make new ones.

Pasteurization also typically leaves the food or beverage with a residual caramelized flavor due to the conversation of many flavinoids and sugars to other compounds. In milk, for example, there is a substantial conversion from lactose to lactulose after UHT pasteurization. Lactulose can cause intestinal cramping, nausea and vomiting.

As for irradiation, there is little research on the resulting nutrient content outside of a few microwave studies (that showed decreased nutrient content and the formation of undesirable metabolites), but there is some evidence that irradiation may denature protein and nutrient molecules.

Whole foods in nature's packages are significantly different from pasteurized processed foods. Fresh whole foods produced by plants contain various antioxidants and enzymes that reduce the ability of microorganisms to grow. The Creator also provided whole foods with peels and shells that protect nutrients and keep most microorganisms out. Microorganisms may invade the outer shell or peel somewhat, but the peel's pH, dryness and density—together with the acidity of the inner fruit—work as a barrier to most microorganisms. For this reason, most fruits and nuts can be easily stored for days and weeks without having significant microbiological risk. Once the peel or shell is removed, the inner fruit, juice or nut must be eaten quickly to prevent contamination, depending upon the fruit's sugar content.

Whole natural foods also contain polysaccharides and oligosaccharides that combine nutrients and sugar within large molecules. These complex molecules are often difficult for pathogenic bacteria to break them down for food. Once processing takes place, however, the sugars are broken down into more simplified form, allowing microbial growth. Why? Because simple sugars provide convenient food and energy sources to growing bacteria and fungi colonies. This means processed food becomes open to mass colonization by microorganisms.

As for milk and milk products, raw milk will contain a number of probiotics that mother cow produces to keep the milk balanced and wholesome. Just as they balance our body's microbiotic content, the probiotics in milk will typically prevent microorganism overgrowth and infection. Still, raw milk should be purchased with caution. Raw milk should only be purchased from certified organic dairies that test for pathogenic microbes. The dairy should also be primarily grass-fed rather than grain-fed. An organic grass-fed cow is less prone to many diseases because eating fresh grass helps prevent disease—just as fresh, raw foods help prevent disease in humans.

Is it the Germ or the Field?

Our bacteria paranoia began in the 1860s with Louis Pasteur's insistence upon the *germ theory*—a proposal that all disease was caused by microorganisms. To prove his point, he cruelly infected various animals with bacteria and studied their demise against uninfected controls. Yes, he proved that bacteria are involved in the pathology of certain diseases, assuming inoculation beyond the capacity of the immune system.

However, he missed a central component of the equation. The fact is our entire planet is covered with infectious microorganisms in numbers beyond calculation. Each human body contains trillions of bacteria. So if the outside and inside world is covered with bacteria, why aren't all of us sick and infected perpetually? How could some of us be healthy with so many microbes around? And how could humans have survived this massive infestation of microbes for so many thousands of years?

Microbiologists Antoine Bechamp and Claude Bernard, peers of Pasteur, took issue with Pasteur's germ theory. They proposed the important issue in disease is not the germ, but the *field*, or environment within the body. Those who get sick, Bechamp and Bernard proposed, were those with weakened and compromised immune systems.

In other words, a healthy body with a strong immune system and healthy probiotic populations is significantly more likely to counter and defeat infective microbes.

We can confirm the field theory quite simply. Foodborne outbreaks result in the sickness and death of only a few people— when thousands, even hundreds of thousands, may actually have consumed the contaminated products.

In fact, many of our foods typically contain *E. coli*, *Salmonella* and many other bacteria species, and do not make people sick.

Unfortunately, Pasteur's germ theory prevailed, and this helped unleash the genie of antibiotics and so many other pharmaceutical panaceas over the last century. While many of these medicines have helped millions resolve infections (after their immune systems recovered), the over-prescription of antibiotics has also destroyed internal probiotic populations and created numerous superbugs more powerful than the previous species of bacteria. In other words, the germ theory solution has created more deadly germs!

The Probiotic Discovery

The pace of the industrial revolution and the progression towards chemical medicine ignored the discoveries that proved the field theory and disproved the germ theory. In the first decade of the twentieth century, Ilya Ilyich Mechnikov, a Nobel Prize-winning (1908) microbiologist, associated the longevity of the Bulgarian and Balkan peoples, and others, with the drinking of fermented milks of cows, buffalos and even reindeers. After years of research, he proposed that there were tiny microorganisms that were living in the fermented milks, and these were somehow stimulating the immune system. He worked with these microorganisms for many years, and also, ironically, worked with Louis Pasteur. His discoveries on the immune system led to our understanding of white blood cells and their ability to phagotize (break apart) invading microbes.

In essence, it was his combination of discoveries that illustrated that infectious microorganisms can be managed and controlled by probiotic organisms that work in cooperation with the immune system. Over the past century since these discoveries, many researchers have followed in Mechnikov's footsteps to find more species and strains of probiotics that live not only within humans, but also within other animals and other environments. Truly, the field theory was proven without a doubt.

In other words, those with healthy immune systems and probiotic populations will typically not get sick from eating a limited amount of contaminated foods. Our bodies typically already contain *E. coli* and *Salmonella*. *E. coli* is often residing in a healthy intestinal tract. Why do we not get sick from these bacteria then? It is because our probiotic bacteria populations keep *E. coli* populations from growing too large. Probiotics produce their own array of antibiotic substances, which inhibit or control pathogenic microorganism populations. The table below summarizes results of two laboratory studies and a review of the research (Chaitow and Trenev 1990) measuring the inhibition zone (or killing distance) three probiotic strains have upon selected pathogenic bacteria:

Bacteria Inhibition by Selected Probiotics

Pathogen	L. acidophilus[1]	L. bulgaricus[2]	B. bifidum[3]
Escherichia coli	44mm	40mm	20mm
Clostridium botulinum	37mm	38mm	not tested
Clostridium perfringens	31mm	33mm	not tested
Proteus mirabilis	39mm	45mm	not tested
Salmonella enteridis	42mm	39mm	not tested
Salmonella typhimurium	44mm	39mm	not tested
Salmonella typhosa	not tested	not tested	12mm
Shigella dysenteriae	30mm	not tested	11mm
Shigella paradysenteriae	30mm	not tested	not tested
Staphylococcus aureus	35mm	38mm	23mm
Staphylococcus faecalis	31mm	39mm	not tested
Bacillus cereus	not tested	not tested	22mm
Pseudomonas fluorescens	not tested	not tested	18mm
Mocrococcus flavis	not tested	not tested	25mm

1. Laboratory tests on *Lactobacillus acidophilus* secretion acidophilin DDS1 adapted from Fernandes *et al.* 1988.
2. Laboratory tests on *Lactobacillus* bulgaricus DDS14 secretion bulgarican adapted from Fernandes *et al.* 1988.
3. Laboratory tests on *Bifidobacterium bifidum* 1452 adapted from Anand *et al.* 1984.

Like animals in the forest, bacteria colonies tend to control each other's populations. In a healthy body and natural environment, our bodies harbor enough probiotics with their own antimicrobial strategies to keep most microorganisms from overgrowth. Our body's probiotics comprise about 70% of our immune response. As we will see in the following chapters, probiotic colonies work with the body's immune system to stimulate an array of antibodies and immune cells that identify and break down infectious microorganisms.

The Living Immune System

When a heart is removed from a dead body and put into a living body, the living body's immune system immediately begins to reject it. This is because the living immune system recognizes this heart as not part of the natural body.

The immune system is located throughout the body. We find immune cells on the skin, in the blood, in the lungs, in the bones and in every organ system. We also find the immune system within trillions of probiotic bacteria scattered around the body.

The immune system has a number of intelligent abilities. The first is recognition. The immune system has the facility to recognize molecules that endanger the body's welfare. The immune system also maintains memory. The immune system can remember the identity of a toxin or pathogen by virtue of recognizing its antigens (byproducts or molecular structure). This is the rationale for vaccination. Vaccination exposes the body to a small amount of a particular pathogen so the immune system will develop the tools and the memory to recognize its antigens, so that the body can respond appropriately the next time it is exposed to the same pathogen.

The immune system is incredible in its ability to maintain specificity and diversity. These characteristics allow the immune system to respond to literally millions, if not billions of different antigens. Moreover, each particular antigen requires a completely different response.

The immune system is an intelligent scanning and review system intended to gauge whether a particular molecule, cell or organism belongs in the body. This is determined through a complex biochemical identification system. We might compare this system to an iris scan, often used as a password entry system. Utilizing a database of information, the immune system checks molecular structures against this database. If the molecu-

33

lar structure isn't recognized, or matches a structure considered foreign, the immune system launches an attack. This attack is referred to as an immune response or an inflammatory response.

Despite significant research in the areas of vaccination, antibiotics, and inflammation, modern medical science is still perplexed with the autoimmune syndrome. A massive list of degenerative diseases are now considered autoimmune, including irritable bowel syndrome, Crohn's, asthma, allergies, fibromyalgia, lupus, urinary tract disorders and many, many others. Physicians also classify most types of arthritis as autoimmune disorders. Why can't the immune system repair these disorders, as it does with most other types of injuries? What has gone wrong with the immune system?

As far as infections go, harmful microbes or chemical toxins invade the body via the digestive tract, the nose and sinuses, the genitals, the lungs, the skin, the ears and even the eyes. Microbial infections can also be caused by normal residents of the body, should they grow beyond their typical populations. These include *H. pylori, E. coli* and *Candida albicans*.

There are four processes the body uses to prevent infection by toxins:

Non-specific Immunity

The first is called the *non-specific* immune response. This utilizes a network of biochemical barriers that work synergistically to prevent infectious agents from getting into the body. The barrier structures include the ability of the body to shut down its orifices. We can close our eyes, mouths, noses and ears to prevent invaders or toxins from entering the body. Within these lie further defensive structures: Nose hairs, eyelashes, lips, tonsils, ear hair, pubic hair and hair in general are all designed to help screen out and filter invaders. Most of the body's passageways are also equipped with tiny cilia, which assist the body evacuate invaders by brushing them out. These cilia move rhythmically, sweeping back and forth, working caught pathogens outward with their undulations. The surfaces of most of the body's orifices are also covered with a mucous membrane. This thin liquid membrane film contains a combination of biochemicals and cells that prevent invaders from penetrating any further. These mucous membranes lining the passageways accomplish this with a combination of immune cells, immunoglobulins and colonies of probiotics.

The digestive tract is equipped with another type of sophisticated defense technology. Should any foreigners get through the lips, teeth, tongue, hairs, mucous membranes, cilia and sneak down the esophagus, they then must contend with the digestive fire of the stomach. The gastrin, peptic acid and hydrochloric acid within a healthy stomach keep a pH of around two. This is typically enough acidity to kill or significantly damage many bacteria. However, a person can mistakenly weaken this protective acid by taking antacids or acid-blockers. In this case, the stomach's ability to neutralize pathogens will be handicapped. In addition, a number of microorganisms are accustomed to acidic environments, and still others can tuck away into clumps of food—especially food that has not been chewed well enough.

Humoral Immunity

The second form of immune response involves a highly technical strategic attack that first identifies the invader's weaknesses, followed by a precise and immediate offensive attack to exploit those weaknesses. This is often called humoral immunity. There are more than a billion different types of antibodies, macrophages and other immune cells that are utilized to mobilize and execute specific attack plans. As an immune cell scans a particular invader, it may recognize a particular biomolecular or behavioral weakness within the toxin or pathogen. Upon recognizing this weakness, the immune system will devise a unique plan to exploit this weakness. It may launch a variety of possible attacks, using a combination of specialized B-cells (or *B-lymphocytes*) in conjunction with specialized antibodies.

Cruising through the blood and lymph systems, the antibodies and/or B-cells can quickly sense and size up invading microbes. Often this will mean the antibody will lock onto or bind to the invader to extract critical genetic information. This process will often draw upon databases held within certain helper B-cells that memorize vulnerabilities. The specific vulnerability is often revealed by molecular structures of pathogenic cell membranes. Each pathogen will be identified by these unique structures or antigens. The B-cell then reproduces a specific antibody designed to record and communicate that information to other B-cells through biochemical transception. This allows for a constant tracking of the location and development of pathogens, allowing B-cells to manage and constantly assess the response.

Cell-Mediated Immunity

The third process used by the immune system is the cell-mediated immune response. This also incorporates a collection of smart white blood cells, called T-cells. T-cells and their surrogates wander the body scanning the body's own cells. They are seeking cells that have become infected or otherwise damaged by microbes or toxic free radicals. Infected cells are typically identified by special marker molecules (antigens) that sit atop their cell membranes. These antigens have particular molecular arrangements that signal roving T-cells of the damage that has occurred within the cell. Once a damaged cell has been recognized, the cell-mediated immune system will launch an inflammatory response against the cell. This response will typically utilize a variety of cytotoxic (cell-killing) cells and helper T-cells. These types of immune cells will often directly kill the damaged cell by inserting toxic chemicals into it. Alternatively, the T-cell might send signals into the damaged cell, switching on a self-destruct mechanism within the cell.

Probiotic Immunity

The fourth and most powerful part of the immune system takes place among the body's probiotics. The human body can house more than 32 billion beneficial and harmful bacteria and fungi at any particular time. When beneficial bacteria are in the majority, they constitute up to 70-80% of the body's immune response. This takes place both in an isolated manner and in conjunction with the rest of the immune system.

Probiotic colonies work with the body's internal immune system to organize strategies that prevent toxins and pathogenic microorganisms from harming the body. Probiotics will communicate and cooperate with the immune system to organize cooperative strategies. They will stimulate the body's immune cells, activating the cell-mediated response, the humoral response, and indirectly, the body's exterior barrier mechanisms through immunoglobulin stimulation. As we will see in the research, they stimulate T-cells, B-cells, macrophages and NK-cells with smart messages that promote specific immune responses. They also activate cytokines and phagocytic cells directly to coordinate their intelligent immune response.

Probiotics can also quickly identify harmful bacteria or fungal overgrowths and work directly to eradicate them. This process may not directly involve the rest of the immune system. Even still, the immune system will be notified of any probiotic offensives. The immune system will support the process by breaking up and escorting dead pathogens out of the body.

Probiotics produce chemical substances that destroy invading microorganisms. Probiotics make up our body's own antibiotic system. Because probiotics are extremely intelligent and want to survive, they have developed various strategies to defend their homeland (our body). It is a territorial issue. Invading bacteria threaten their homes and families. Probiotics also learn how to fight newer bacteria species and new bacteria strategies. While static pharmaceutical antibiotics are counteracted by smart super-bugs, probiotics can alter their antibiotic strategies as needed. Our continued survival illustrates their intelligence.

Probiotics produce antimicrobial biochemicals that manage, damage or kill pathogenic microorganisms. In some cases, they will simply overcrowd the invaders with biochemistry and populations to limit their growth. In other cases, they will secrete chemicals into the fluid environment to eradicate large populations. In still other cases, they will insert specific chemicals into the invaders, which will directly kill them. Probiotic mechanisms are quite complex and variegated to say the least.

Dr. Mechnikov hypothesized that the beneficial effects of lactobacilli arise from the lactic acid they excrete. Indeed, the lactic acid produced by *Lactobacillus* and *Bifidobacteria* species sets up the ultimate pH control in the gut to repel antagonistic organisms. Lactic acids are not alike, however. There are different lactic acid molecular structures, and combinations with other chemicals. For example, some probiotics produce an L(+) form of lactic acid and other probiotics may produce the D(-) from. Many probiotic strains also produce a molecular combination with hydrogen peroxide called lactoperoxidase.

Probiotics also produce acetic acids, formic acids lipopolysaccharides, peptidoglycans, superantigens, heat shock proteins and bacterial DNA—all in precise portions to nourish each other, inhibit challengers and/or benefit the host.

Precision and proportion is the key. For example, some bifidobacteria secrete a 3:2 proportion of acetic acid to lactic acid in order to barricade certain pathogenic microbes.

Probiotics also secrete a number of key nutrients crucial to its host's (our body) immune system and metabolism, including B vitamins pantothenic acid, pyridoxine, niacin, folic acid, cobalamin and biotin, and crucial antioxidants such as vitamin K.

Probiotics also produce antimicrobial molecules called bacteriocins. *Lactobacillus plantarum* produces lactolin. *Lactobacillus bulgaricus* secretes bulgarican. *Lactobacillus acidophilus* can produce aciophilin, acidolin, bacterlocin and lactocidin. These and other antimicrobial substances equip probiotic species with territorial mechanisms to combat and reduce pathologies related to *Shigella, Coliform, Pseudomonas, Klebsiella, Staphylococcus, Clostridium, Escherichia* and other infective genera. Furthermore, antifungal biochemicals from the likes of *L. acidophilus, B. bifidum, E. faecium* and others also significantly reduce fungal outbreaks caused by *Candida albicans* (Shahani *et al.* 2005).

These types of antimicrobial tools give probiotics the ability to counter the mighty *H. pylori* bacterium—known to be at the root of a majority of ulcers. *H. pylori* inhibition has been observed in studies on *L. acidophilus* DDS-1, *L. rhamnosus* GG, *L. rhamnosus Lc705, Propionibacterium freudenreichii* and *Bifidobacterium breve Bb99,* as we will see later.

Furthermore, probiotics will specifically stimulate the body's own immune system to attack pathogens. For example, scientists from Finland's University of Turku (Pessi *et al.* 2000) gave nine atopic dermatitis children *Lactobacillus rhamnosus* GG for four weeks. They found that serum cytokine IL-10 levels specific to the infection increased following probiotic consumption.

Whatever the strategy, smart probiotic microorganisms work collectively and synergistically with the other three components of our immune system. Our probiotic system works within the non-specific immune system to help protect the body from invasions. Probiotics live within the oral cavity, the nasal cavity, the esophagus, around the gums, and in pockets of our pleural cavity (surrounding our lungs). They dwell within our stomach, within our intestines, within the vagina and around the rectum, and amongst other pockets of tissues. This means that for microbes to invade the bloodstream, they must first get through legions of probiotic bacteria that populate those entry channels— assuming a healthy body of course.

In order to better understand the relationship between probiotics and our immune system, let's discuss the other players among the body's immune system and their interaction with our probiotic populations.

White Blood Cells

The immune system produces at least five different types of white blood cells. Each is designed to identify and target specific types of pathogens. After identification, they will either initiate an attack with other components, or directly begin their attack. The main types are lymphocytes, neutrophils, basophils, monocytes and macrophages. Each plays an important role in the pathogen-identification and inflammatory process. Lymphocytes are the body's self-specific immune response team.

The primary lymphocytes are the T-cells (thymus cells) or B-cells (bone marrow cells). These cells and their specialized proteins work together to strategically attack and remove invaders. Then they memorize the strategy in preparation for a future invasion.

All white blood cells are initially assembled by stem cells in the bone marrow. Following their release, T-cells undergo further differentiation and programming in the thymus gland. B-cells undergo a similar process of maturity before release from the spleen. Both T-cells and B-cells circulate via lymph nodes, the bloodstream and among tissue fluids. Both also have a number of special types, including memory cells and helper cells to identify and memorize invaders.

B-cells look for foreign or potentially harmful pathogens moving freely. These might include toxins or microbes. Once identified, B-cells will stimulate the production of a particular type of antibody protein, which is designed to destroy or break apart the foreigner. There are several different types of B-cells. Most are monoclonal, which means they will adjust to the specific type of invader. Some B-cells are investigative and surveillance oriented. They are focused on roaming pathogens. Once activated, they can then damage these invading pathogens using a variety of biochemical secretions or physical activities. B-cells that circulate and surveil the bloodstream are often called plasma B-cells. Others—like memory B-cells—record previous invasions for future attacks.

T-cells, on the other hand, are oriented toward the body's own cells. They are focused upon internal cellular problems, toxin absorption, or those pathogens that have invaded cells.

There are different types of T-cells. Each is programmed in the thymus to look for a different type of problem, and each has the capability of destroying different types of cells and infections. Many T-cells simply respond to a pathogen that has invaded the cell by destroying the cell itself—this is the *killer* T-cell. It does this by inserting special chemicals into the cell or submitting instructions for the cell to kill itself. Cell death is called apoptosis, and T-cells capable of killing our cells are called cytotoxic T-cells and natural killer T-cells.

T-cells work through a communication system of cytokines to relay instructions and information amongst the various T-cells. Prominent cytokine communications thus take place between helper T-cells, natural killer cells and cytotoxic T-cells.

The initial scanning of an infected cell by a helper T-cell utilizes electromagnetic scanning just as the B-cells do. The T-cell's support network also includes delta-gamma T-cells. Delta-gamma T-cells are stimulated by specific molecular receptors on cell membranes. In general, helper T-cells communicate previous immune responses, memorize current ones, and pass on strategic information on the progress of pending attack plans.

The helper T-cell scan surveys the cell's membrane for indications of either microbial infection or some sort of genetic mutation due to a virus or toxin. This antigen scan might reveal invasions of chemical toxins, protozoa, worms, fungi, bacteria and viruses that have intruded or deranged the cell. The scanning helper T-cell immediately communicates the information by releasing their tiny coded protein cytokines. These disseminate the information needed to coordinate macrophages, NK-cells and cytotoxic T-cells for attack.

Probiotics participate in these communications. In one study, the probiotic organism *Bifidobacterium lactis* HN019 or a placebo was given to 30 healthy elderly volunteers (average age 69 years old) for nine weeks. The probiotic group had significant increases among total T-cells, helper T-cells (CD4+), activated (CD25+) T-cells, and natural killer T-cells. Cytotoxic capacity among mononuclear and polymorphonuclear phagocytes and tumor-cell killing activity among natural killer cells also increased among the probiotic group (Gill *et al.* 2001).

Most cells contain tumor necrosis factor or TNF—a sort of self-destruct switch. When signaled from the outside by a T-cell, TNF will initiate a self-destruct and the cell will die.

Under some circumstances, entire groups of cells or tissue systems may be damaged. Macrophages may be signalled to cut off the blood supply to kill these deranged or infected cells.

The two primary helper T-cell types are the Th1 and the Th2. The Th1 T-cell focuses on the elimination of bacteria, fungi, parasites, viruses, and similar types of invaders. The Th2 cells, on the other hand, are focused upon allergic and antibody responses. The Th2 is thus explicitly involved in the responses of inflammation and allergic reaction. This is important to note, because research has revealed that stress, chemical toxins, poor dietary habits and lack of sleep tend to suppress Th1 levels and increase Th2 levels. With an abundance of Th2 cells in the system, the body is prone to respond more strongly to allergens and toxins, causing problems like hay fever and allergies. This is also why we sometimes see people who are under physical or emotional stress overreacting with hives, psoriasis and other allergic-type responses.

Probiotics modulate the Th1/Th2 system. Illustrating this, yogurt with *Bifidobacterium longum* BB536 or plain yogurt was given to 40 patients with Japanese cedar pollinosis for 14 weeks.

Peripheral blood mononuclear cells from the patients indicated that *B. fragilis* microorganisms induced significantly more helper TH cell type2 cytokines such as interleukin [IL]-6, and fewer Th1 cytokines such as IL-12 and interferon (Odamaki *et al.* 2007).

Neutrophils are white blood cells that circulate within the blood stream, looking for abnormal behavior among various cells and tissues. Once they identify a problem, they will signal a mass assembly and begin the process of cleaning the area. This typically involves inflammation, as they work to break down and remove debris.

Neutrophils are also coordinated by probiotics. Researchers from the Liver Failure Group and The Institute of Hepatology at the University College London's Medical School (Stadlbauer *et al.* 2008) found in a study of 20 liver failure patients that neutrophil function and cytokines were significantly modulated by the probiotic *Lactobacillus casei* Shirota. Starting neutrophil phagocytic capacity was significantly lower than healthy controls (73% versus 98%) before probiotic treatment. Neutrophil phagocytic capacity after probiotic treatments were equal between the cirrhosis patients and the healthy volunteers at the end of the study—while the placebo group's neutrophil capacity did not change. In addition, endotoxin-stimulated TNF-receptors 1 and 2 and interleukin-10 (IL-10) levels were significantly lower among the probiotic group. The scientists concluded: "Our data provide a proof-of-concept that probiotics restore neutrophil phagocytic capacity in cirrhosis, possibly by changing IL10 secretion and TLR4 expression."

Monocytes are like the neolithic ancestors of the attack soldiers. After being produced in the marrow, monocytes differentiate into either macrophages or dendrite cells. The macrophages are particularly good at engulfing and breaking apart pathogens. Dendritic cells are interactive cells that stimulate certain responses. They may, for example, isolate and present a pathogen to the T-cells. Dendritic cells also stimulate the production of those special inter-white blood cell communication proteins called cytokines.

Probiotics utilize cytokine communications to transmit intelligent information to the body's network of white blood cells. Illustrating this, Scientists from the Slovak Institute of Cardiovascular Diseases (Hlivak *et al.* 2005) gave a placebo or probiotic *Enterococcus faecium* M-74 to human volunteers for 60 weeks. Peripheral blood analysis indicated significant decreases in cytokines sICAM-1, CD54 on monocytes, and CD11b on lymphocytes after one-year. These are related to anti-adhesion strategies following inflammatory responses to artery damage.

In another study, researchers from Poland's Pomeranian Academy of Medicine (Naruszewicz *et al.* 2002) gave *Lactobacillus plantarum* 299v or placebo to 36 healthy (but smoker) volunteers for six weeks. Monocytes isolated from probiotic subjects had significantly reduced adhesion to endothelial cells, and the probiotic group had significant decreases in systolic blood pressure, leptin levels, and fibrinogen levels. The probiotic group also had a 42% reduction in cytokine interleukin-6. No changes were observed among the placebo group.

Cytokines

As mentioned, cytokines are communication devices that allow different immune cells to communicate. These typically come with complex names like interleukin (IL), transforming growth factor (TGF), leukemia inhibitory factor (LIF), and tumor necrosis factor (TNF). There are five basic types of cell communication: intracrine, autocrine, endocrine, juxtacrine and paracrine.

Autocrine communication takes place between two different types of cells. This message can be a biochemical exchange or an electromagnetic signal. The other cell in turn may respond automatically by producing a particular biochemical or electromagnetic message. We might compare this to leaving a voicemail on someone's message machine. Once we leave the message, the machine signals that the message has been received and will be delivered. Later the machine will replay the message. The immune system uses this type of autocrine message recording process to activate T-cells. Once the message is relayed, the T-cell will respond specifically with the instructed activity.

A paracrine communication takes place between neighboring cells of the same type, to pass on a message that comes from outside of the tissue system. Tiny protein antennas will sit on cell membranes, allowing one cell to communicate with another. This allows cells within the same tissue system to respond in a coordinated manner.

Juxtacrine communications take place via smart biomolecular structures. We might call these structures relay stations. They absorb messages and pass them on. An example of this is the passing of inflammatory messages via immune cell cytokines.

An intracrine communication takes place within the cell. First, an external message may be communicated into the cell through an antenna sitting on the cell's membrane. Once inside the cell, the message will be communicated around cell's organelles to initiate internal metabolic responses.

The endocrine message takes place between endocrine glands and individual cells. The endocrine glands include the pineal gland, the pituitary gland, the pancreas, adrenals, thyroid, ovary and testes. These glands produce endocrine biochemicals, which relay messages directly to cells. Their messages stimulate a variety of metabolic functions within the body. These include growth, temperature, sexual behavior, sleep, glucose utilization, stress response and so many others. One of the functions of the endocrine glands relevant to disease is the production of inflammatory co-factors such as cortisol, adrenaline and norepinephrine. These coordinate and initiate instructions that stimulate inflammatory processes.

Probiotics also utilize these systems to communicate with the body's various cells. They utilize paracrine and juxtacrine communications to pass on messages about the location, type and weaknesses of invading organisms. These messages are then compared with the programmed history within helper T-cells and helper B-cells. This creates a coordinated response. For example, the immune system might launch phagocytic cells to help attack the pathogens a probiotic colony may be battling.

Scientists from the Nagoya University Graduate School of Medicine's Department of Surgery (Sugawara *et al.* 2006) found in a study of 101 patients that supplementation with probiotics increased NK activity and lymphocyte counts. Pro-inflammatory IL-6 cytokines decreased significantly among the probiotic group. Serum IL-6, white blood cell counts, and C-reactive protein also significantly decreased among the probiotic group.

Furthermore, probiotics have the ability to *uniquely modify* cytokines depending upon the condition and disease of the person. Illustrating this, a probiotic drink with either placebo or a probiotic combination of *Lactobacillus paracasei* Lpc-37, *Lactobacillus acidophilus* 74-2 and *Bifidobacterium animalis* subsp. *lactis* DGCC 420 (*B. lactis* 420) was given to 15 healthy adults and 15 adults with atopic dermatitis. After 8 weeks, CD57(+) cytokines levels increased significantly among the healthy group taking probiotics, while CD4(+)CD54(+) cytokines decreased significantly among the AD patients who were taking the probiotics, compared with the placebo group and compared to the levels at the beginning of the trial (Roessler *et al.* 2008).

Inflammatory Stimulators

Our body's immune system launches inflammatory cells and factors that heal injury sites and prevent bleed-outs. This process is often stimulated by leukotrienes and prostaglandins.

Leucotrienes are molecules that identify problems and stimulate the immune system. They pinpoint and isolate areas of the body that require repair. Once they pinpoint the site of repair, one type of leucotriene will initiate inflammation, and others will assist in maintaining the process. Once the repair process proceeds to a point of maturity, another type of leucotriene will begin slowing down the process of inflammation.

This smart signalling process takes place through the biochemical bonding formations of these molecules. Leucotrienes are paracrines and autocrines. They are paracrine in that they initiate messages that travel from one cell to another. They are autocrine in that they initiate messages that encourage an automatic and immediate response—notably among T-cells, engaging them to remove bad cells. They also help transmit messages that initiate the process of repair through the clotting of blood and the patching of damaged tissues.

Leucotrienes are produced from the conversion of essential fatty acids (EFAs) by an enzyme produced by the body called arachidonate-5-lipoxygenase (sometimes called LOX). The central fatty acids of this process are arachidonic acid (AA), gammalinolenic acid (GLA), and eicosapentaenoic acid (EPA). Lipoxygenase enzymes produce different types of leucotrienes, depending upon the initial fatty acid. The important point of this is that the leucotrienes produced by arachidonic acid stimulate inflammation, while the leucotrienes produced by EPA halt inflammation. The leucotrienes produced by GLA, on the other hand, block the conversion process of polyunsaturated fatty acids to arachidonic acid.

Prostaglandins are also produced through an enzyme conversion from fatty acids. Like leucotrienes, prostaglandins are messengers that transmit particular messages to immune cells. Their messaging is either paracrine or autocrine. Prostaglandins are critical parts of the process of injury repair. They also initiate a number of protective sequences in the body, including the transmission of pain and the clotting of blood.

Prostaglandins are produced by the oxidation of fatty acids by an enzyme produced in the body called cyclooxygenase—also called prostaglandin-endoperoxide synthase (PTGS) or COX.

There are three types of COX, and each convert fatty acids to different types of prostaglandins. The central fatty acid that causes inflammation again is arachidonic acid. COX-1 converts AA to the PGE2 type of prostaglandin. COX-2, on the other hand, converts AA into the PGI2 type of prostaglandin.

The central messages that prostaglandins transmit depend upon the type of prostaglandin. Prostaglandin I2 (also PGI2) stimulates the widening of blood vessels and bronchial passages, and pain sensation within the nervous system. In other words, along with stimulating blood clotting, PGI2 signals a range of responses to assist the body's wound healing at the site of injury.

Prostaglandin E2, or PGE2, is altogether different from PGI2. PGE2 stimulates the secretion of mucus within the stomach, intestines, mouth and esophagus. It also decreases the production of gastric acid in the stomach. This combination of increasing mucus and lowering acid production keeps healthy stomach cells from being damaged by our gastric acids and the acidic content of our foods. This is one of the central reasons NSAID pharmaceuticals cause gastrointestinal problems: They interrupt the secretion of this protective mucus in the stomach.

This means that the COX-1 enzyme instigates the process of protecting the stomach, while the COX-2 enzyme instigates the process of inflammation and repair within the body. In the case of autoimmune disease, the COX-2 process often lies at the root of pain and swelling.

Cyclooxygenase also converts ALA/DHA and GLA to prostaglandins. Just as lipoxygenase converts ALA/DHA and GLA to anti-inflammation leucotrienes, the conversion of ALA/DHA and GLA by cyclooxygenase produces prostaglandins that either block the inflammatory process or reverse it. This means that a healthy diet with plenty of GLA and ALA/DHA fats will balance inflammation response. ALA is found in walnuts, soybeans, flax, canola, pumpkin seeds and chia seeds. The purest form of DHA is found in certain algae, and the body produces EPA from DHA.

Fish and krill also get their DHA up the food chain from algae. GLA is found in borage, primrose oil and spirulina.

Probiotics are often involved in the production of intermediary fatty acids used for these LOX and COX conversions, producing anti-inflammatory effects. To illustrate this, scientists from the University of Helsinki (Kekkonen *et al.* 2008) measured lipids and inflammation markers before and after giving probiotic *Lactobacillus rhamnosus* GG to 26 healthy adults. After three weeks of probiotic supplementation, the subjects had decreased levels of intermediary inflammatory fatty acids such as lysophosphatidylcholines, sphingomyelins, and several glycerophosphatidylcholines. Probiotics also reduced inflammatory markers TNF-alpha and CRP in this study.

The arachidonic acid conversion process that produces prostaglandins also produces thromboxanes. Thromboxanes stimulate platelets in the blood to aggregate. They work in concert with platelet-activating factor or PAF. Together, these biomolecules drive the process of clotting the blood and restricting blood flow. This is good during injury healing, but the inflammatory process must also be slowed down as the injury heals.

Probiotics help modulate that process. In the research from Poland's Pomeranian Academy of Medicine (Naruszewicz *et al.* 2002) mentioned earlier, scientists found that giving *Lactobacillus plantarum* 299v to 36 volunteers resulted in a 37% decrease in inflammatory F2-isoprostanes. Isoprostanes are similar to prostaglandins, formed outside of the COX process.

Immunoglobulins

Immunoglobulins are proteins that are programmed for a particular type of response in the presence of particular pathogens in different areas and maturity. IgA immunoglobulins line the mouth and digestive tract, scanning for pathogens that might infect the body. IgDs sense infections and activate B-cells. IgEs attach to foreign substances and launch histamine responses—

typically associated with allergic responses. IgGs cross through membranes, responding to growing pathogens that have already invaded the body. IgMs are focused on new intrusions that have yet to grow enough to garner the attention of the IgGs.

Each of these general immunoglobulin categories contain numerous sub-types geared to different types of pathogens and responses. Other immunoglobulin proteins also exist. Some of these aid macrophages and lymphocytes in identifying specific pathogens.

An element of immunoglobulins is the CD glycogen-protein complex. CD stands for cluster of differentiation. CDs are molecules that sit on top of immune cells to navigate and steer their behavior. They will sit atop T-cells, B-cells, NK-cells, granulocytes and monocytes, identifying pathogens and infected cells. They often negotiate and bind to pathogens. This allows the lymphocyte to proceed to attack the pathogen, often by inserting a toxic chemical that destroys the pathogen or the cell hosting it.

CDs are identified by their molecular structure: This is also referred to as a ligand. The specific molecular arrangement (or CD number) will also match a specific type of receptor at the membrane of the cell or pathogen. Each CD number will produce a bonding relationship with a certain receptor structure on the cell to allow the accompanying immunoglobulin or lymphocyte to have interactivity with the pathogen. This gives the immunoglobulin or lymphocyte an access point from which to attack the pathogen.

Immunoglobulins and CDs are also tools probiotics utilize to define or influence appropriate responses for the immune system. Probiotics stimulate IgAs through CDs, for example, when they discover a pathogen has invaded parts of the body's entry passageways.

CDs are also utilized by probiotics to define the cells and tissue systems that have been damaged by toxins, bacteria, or viruses. Probiotics will respond appropriately, signalling back and forth with the immune system. This signalling often stimulates particular inflammatory and injury-healing responses.

Illustrating this, Finnish scientists (Ouwehand *et al.* 2009) gave healthy elderly volunteers lactitol (a milk sugar) with *Lactobacillus acidophilus* or a placebo. The group given the probiotics showed a significant modification of pro-inflammatory IgA and PGE2 levels. The researchers also noticed that levels of bifidobacteria in the stool of the elderly subjects were similar to those of a young person—as usually bifidobacteria colonies are reduced among the elderly. They also observed improved spermidine levels—an enzyme involved in DNA synthesis. These improvements suggested increased mucosal and intestinal immunity and probiotic content among the probiotic group.

In a study of 105 pregnant women, University of Western Australia scientists (Prescott *et al.* 2008) found that *Lactobacillus rhamnosus* and *Bifidobacterium lactis* stimulated higher levels of cytokine IFN-gamma, higher levels of TGF-beta1, and higher levels of breast milk IgA. Plasma of their babies had lower CD14 levels, and greater CB IFN-gamma levels. These indicated improvements in immune response stimulated by the probiotics.

In another example, researchers from the Turku University Central Hospital in Finland (Rinne *et al.* 2005) gave 96 mothers either a placebo or *Lactobacillus rhamnosus* GG before delivery and continued the supplementation in their infants after delivery. At three months of age, immunoglobulin IgG-secreting cells among breastfed infants supplemented with probiotics were significantly higher than the breastfed infants who received the placebo. In addition, IgM-, IgA-, and IgG-secreting cell counts at 12 months were significantly higher among the breastfed infants who supplemented with probiotics, compared to breastfed infants receiving the placebo.

In yet another example, researchers from the Teikyo University School of Medicine in Japan (Araki *et al.* 1999) gave *Bifidobacterium breve* YIT4064 or placebo to 19 infants for 28 days.

Rotavirus shedding in the feces of the probiotic group was significantly reduced compared to the placebo group. IgA levels also significantly changed among the probiotic group.

Inflammation

Inflammation coordinates the various immune players into a frenzy of healing. Imagine for a moment cutting your finger pretty badly. First you would feel pain—letting you know the body is hurt and to pay attention to it. Second, you will probably notice that the area has become swollen and red. Blood starts to clot around the spot. Soon the cut stops bleeding. The blood dries and a scab forms. It remains red, maybe a little hot, and hurts for a while. After the healing proceeds, soon the cut is closed up and there is a scab left with a little redness around it. The pain soon stops. The scab falls off and the finger returns to normal—almost like new and ready for reuse.

Without this inflammatory process, we might not even know we cut our finger in the first place. We might keep working, only to find out that we had bled out a quart of blood on the floor. Without clotting, it would be hard to stop the bleeding. Were it not for our immune system and inflammatory process slowing blood flow, clotting the blood, scabbing and cleaning up the site, our bodies would simply be full of holes and wounds. We simply could not survive.

We might wonder what this has to do with probiotics. While the body's immune system responds to heal wounds, the body's probiotic system keeps populations of bacteria, fungi and viruses minimized. This prevents infection to the wound by these organisms. If we were to cut our finger whilst our body was overwhelmed with various pathogens like staphylococci and streptococci, for example, the cut could become lethally infected.

The antimicrobial strategy says that an infected wound results from exposure to microbes from the outside environment. This is only partially true. Microbes can also come from within the body. Microbes can be residing in and amongst various tissue systems, and may invade an open wound, where bacteria have access to oxygen. Pathogenic microbes within the body may infect other tissue systems as well. As mentioned, recent research has indicated that the heart and arteries may become infected with bacteria—leading to heart disease and stroke. Joints may become infected—leading to rheumatoid or septic arthritis. The liver may be infected—leading to hepatitis. The stomach may be infected—leading to ulcers. During a systemic or septic infection of *Staphylococcus aureus*, for example, bacteria can necrotize (or kill off) many different cells and tissue systems around the body, including the tissues around open wounds.

The probiotic system and immunoglobulin immune system work together to deter and kill particular invaders—hopefully before they gain access to the body's tissues. Should these defenses fail, they can stimulate the humoral immune system in a strategic attack that includes identifying the pathogens and recognizing their weaknesses. B-cells and probiotics coordinate through the stimulation of immunoglobulins and CDs.

This progression also stimulates an activation of neutrophils, phagocytes, immunoglobulins, leukotrienes and prostaglandins. Should cells become infected, they will signal the immune system from paracrines located on their cell membranes. Once the intrusion and strategy is determined, B-cells will surround the pathogens while T-cells attack any infected cells. Natural killer T-cells may secrete chemicals into infected cells, initiating the death of the cell.

Leukotrienes immediately gather in the region of injury or infection, and signal to T-cells to coordinate efforts in the process of repair. Prostaglandins initiate the widening of blood vessels to bring more T-cells and other repair factors (such as plasminogen and fibrin) to the infected or injured site.

Prostaglandins also stimulate the substance P within the nerve cells, initiating the sensation of pain. At the same time, thromboxanes, along with fibrin, drive the process of clotting and coagulation in the blood, while constricting certain blood vessels to decrease the risk of bleeding.

In the case where the pathogen is an allergen, the inflammation response will also accompany and H1-histamine response. Histamine is primarily produced by the masT-cells and basophils after being stimulated by IgE antibodies. This parallel response serves to help remove the pathogen using physiological responses such as sneezing, watering of the eyes and coughing. These measures, though sometimes considered irritating, are all stimulated in an effort to remove the pathogen and prevent its re-entry into the body. As the H1 histamine binds with receptors, this also encourages alertness (also why antihistamines cause drowsiness). These are the body's natural responses to remove pathogens from the body.

At the height of the repair process, swelling, redness and pain are at their peak. The T-cells, macrophages, neutrophils, fibrin and plasmin all work together to repair the damage. This process is also coordinated with probiotics, who guard against further microbial invasion along the perimeters.

As the process proceeds, the pathogens slowly become be arrested and the damage is repaired. Here macrophages continue the clean up while the other immune cells begin to retreat. Antioxidants like glutathione will attach to and transport the by-products—broken down pathogens and cell parts—out of the body. As this proceeds, both prostaglandins and leucotrienes begin to signal a reversal of the inflammation and pain process.

Probiotics are intimately involved in this normalization process. One of the central features of the normalization process is the production of bradykinin. Bradykinin slows clotting and opens blood vessels to allow the cleanup process to accelerate. A key signalling factor is the production of nitric oxide (NO). NO slows inflammation by promoting the detachment of lymphocytes to the site, and reduces tissue swelling. NO also accelerates

the clearing out of debris with its interaction with the supe......
anion. NO was originally described as endothelium-derived relaxing factor (or EDRF)—because of its role in relaxing blood
vessel walls.

While the body produces nitric oxide in the presence of good
nutrition and lower stress, probiotics also play a big role in nitric
oxide production. Lactobacilli such as *L. plantarum* remove the
harmful nitrate molecule and use it to produce nitric oxide
(Bangmark *et al.* 1998). This is beneficial to not only reducing
inflammation: NO production also creates a healthy environment for metabolism.

Low nitric oxide levels are associated with a plethora of diseases, including diabetes, heart failure, high cholesterol, ulcerative colitis, premature aging, cancers and many others. Low or
abnormal NO production is also seen among lifestyle habits such
as smoking, obesity, and living around air pollution—factors that
also so happen to reduce probiotic colonies.

The Thymus Gland

One of the most important players in the immune system is
the thymus gland. The thymus gland is located in the center of
the chest, behind the sternum. The thymus is one of the more
critical organs of the lymphatic system. Some have compared the
thymus gland of the lymphatic system to the heart of the circula-
tory system.

The thymus gland is not a pump, however. The thymus acti-
vates T-cells and various hormones that modulate and stimulate
the immune and autoimmune processes. The thymus converts a
type of lymphocyte called the thymocyte into T-cells or natural
killer cells. These activated T-cells are released into the lymph
and bloodstream ready to protect and serve. Within the thymus,
the T-cells are infused with CD surface markers—which identify
particular types of problematic cells or invading organisms. The
CD markers define their mission.

In other words, the thymus codes the T-cells with receptors that will bind to particular cells or toxins. The types of cells or toxins they bind to or identify are determined by the major histocompatibility complex, or MHC determinant. During the process of converting thymocytes to T-cells, their receptors are programmed with MHC combinations. This allows them to tolerate particular frailties within the body while attacking what the body considers to be true invaders (Kazansky 2008).

Therefore, it is the MHC that gives the T-cell the ability to identify the difference between *self* and *non-self* parts of the body. A non-self identification will produce an immunogen—a factor that stimulates an immune response. Once the immunogen is processed, it stimulates the inflammatory cascade.

The thymus gland develops and enlarges from birth. It is most productive and at its largest during puberty. From that point on, depending upon our diet, stress and lifestyle, our thymus gland will shrink over the years. By forty, an immunosuppressed person will often have a tiny thymus gland. In elderly persons, the thymus gland is often barely recognizable. For some, the thymus is practically non-functional.

Throughout its productive life, the thymus gland processes T-cells with the appropriate MHC programming. If the thymus gland is functioning, it will continue to produce T-cells with MHC programming that reflects the body's current status. The revised programming will accommodate the various genetic changes that can happen to different cells around the body as we age and adapt to our changing environment. With a shrunken and non-functioning thymus, however, its ability to re-program T-cells with a new MHC—enabling them to identify the body's cells that have adapted—is damaged. The T-cells will have to keep working off the old MHC programming. This means the T-cells will not be able to properly identify self versus non-self.

Herein we find at least part of the solution to the mystery of autoimmune disease.

Probiotics, on the other hand, stimulate a healthy thymus gland. Illustrating this, medical researchers from the University of Bari (Indrio *et al.* 2007) gave a placebo or a probiotic combination of *Bifidobacterium breve* C50 and *Streptococcus thermophilus* 065 to 60 newborns in a randomized, placebo-controlled study on thymus size. Thymus size was significantly larger in the probiotic group compared to the standard formula (placebo) group after the probiotic treatment period.

The Liver

Some call the liver the body's chemical factory. It is really the body's lifeline. The liver sits just below the lungs on the right side under the diaphragm. Partially protected by the ribs, it attaches to the abdominal wall with the falciform ligament. The ligamentum teres within the falciform is the remnant of the umbilical cord that once brought us blood from mama's placenta. As the body develops, the liver continues to filter, purify and enrich our blood. Should the liver shut down, the body would die within hours.

Into the liver drains nutrition-rich venous blood through the hepatic portal vein together with some oxygenated blood through the hepatic artery. A healthy liver will process almost a half-gallon of blood per minute. The blood is commingled within well cavities called sinusoids, where blood is staged through stacked sheets of the liver's primary cells—called hepatocytes. Here blood is also met by interspersed immune cells called kupffers. These kupffer cells attack and break apart bacteria and toxins. Nutrients coming in from the digestive tract are filtered and converted to molecules the body's cells can utilize. The liver also converts old red blood cells to bilirubin to be shipped out of the body. Filtered and purified blood is jettisoned through hepatic veins out the inferior vena cava and back into circulation.

The liver's filtration/purification mechanisms protect our body from various infectious diseases and chemical toxins. After hepatocytes and kuppfer cells break down toxins, the waste is disposed through the gall bladder and kidneys. The gall bladder channels bile from the liver to the intestines. Recycled bile acids combine with bilirubin, phospholipids, calcium and cholesterol to make bile. Bile is concentrated and pumped through the bile duct to the intestines. Here bile acids help digest fats, and broken down toxins are (hopefully) excreted through our feces. Assuming we have healthy probiotic colonies within the intestines.

The liver produces over a thousand biochemicals the body requires for healthy functioning. The liver maintains blood sugar balance by monitoring glucose levels and producing glucose metabolites. It manufactures albumin to maintain plasma pressure. It produces cholesterol, urea, inflammatory biochemicals, blood-clotting molecules, and many others.

Interspersed within the liver are functional fat factories called stellates. These cells store and process lipids, fat-soluble vitamins such as vitamin A, and secrete structural biomolecules like collagen, laminin and glycans. These are used to build some of the body's toughest tissue systems.

We know that our livers become burdened from the avalanche of toxins pelting our bodies. Today our diets, water and air are full of plasticizers, formaldehyde, heavy metals, hydrocarbons, DDT, dioxin, VOCs, asbestos, preservatives, artificial flavors, food dyes, propellants, synthetic fragrances and more. Every single chemical requires the liver to work harder.

Frankly, most livers are now overloaded and beyond their natural capacity. What happens then? Generally, two things. First, the hepatocytes collapse from overtoxification, causing genetic mutation, cell death, and liver exhaustion. Secondly, their weakened condition opens hepatocytes to diseases from infectious agents such as viral hepatitis.

Liver disease—where one or more lobes begin to malfunction—can result in a life-threatening emergency. Cirrhosis is a common diagnosis for liver disease, often caused by years of drinking alcohol or taking prescription medications. During its downfall into cirrhosis, the sub-functioning liver can also cause jaundice, high cholesterol, gallstones, encephalopathy, kidney disease, clotting problems, heart conditions, hormone imbalances and many others. As cirrhosis proceeds, it results in the liver cells' massive die-off and subsequent scarring, causing the liver to begin to shutdown.

While most of us have heard about the damage alcohol can have on the liver, many do not realize that pharmaceuticals and even some supplements can also be extremely toxic to the liver. The liver must find a way to break down these foreign chemicals. Many pharmaceuticals require a Herculean effort simply because the liver's various purification processes were not designed for these foreign molecules. As liver cells weaken and die their enzymes leak into the bloodstream. Blood tests for AST and ALT enzymes can reveal this weakening of the liver.

We must therefore closely monitor the quantity and types of chemicals we put into our body. Eliminating preservatives, food dyes and pesticides in our foods can be done easily by eating whole organic foods. We can eliminate exposures to many environmental toxins mentioned above by simply replacing them with natural alternatives.

A number of herbs help detoxify and strengthen the liver. These include goldenseal, dandelion, milk thistle and others.

Probiotics also play a large role in liver disease. When pathogenic bacteria get out of control in the intestines, they can overload the liver with endotoxins—their waste products. The bombardment of endotoxins onto the liver produces a result similar to alcohol or pharmaceuticals: When complex proteins (such as found in animal products) are putrefied by pathogenic bacteria, one of the metabolites is excessive ammonia. Ammonia is toxic to the liver.

In addition, urea is metabolized by pathogenic bacteria such as *Clostridium* spp., resulting in ammonia and carbon dioxide.

Liver cells are damaged by this onslaught of endotoxins and metabolites produced by pathogenic bacteria.

In a study from scientists at the G.B. Pant Hospital in New Delhi (Sharma *et al.* 2008), 190 cirrhosis patients were given a combination of probiotics for one month. The probiotic group experienced a 51.6% improvement in symptoms, as measured by psychometric testing and blood ammonia levels.

Immune Colonization

To illustrate the general immune effects of probiotics, let's consider the increasing emergence of foodborne *Escherichia coli* outbreaks. *E. coli* is a natural organism living all around us and within our guts. In a healthy body, *E. coli* colonies are heavily outnumbered by colonies of probiotics such as *Lactobacillus acidophilus* and *Bifidus regularis*. These probiotic colonies keep *E. coli* numbers minimized. Should new *E. coli* colonies arrive; probiotics mobilize natural antibiotics to squash and limit the invasion. We consume *E. coli* everyday in so many foods. When we consider how few people get sick, when hundreds of thousands of people have eaten an infected food, we can see how strong of a role probiotic colonization has. Otherwise, how could such a small percentage of the thousands of people who ate an infected packaged food during an outbreak actually get sick?

Furthermore, of those hundreds that may get sick from a massive *E. coli* outbreak, even fewer people actually become *fatally* sick: Very few people will die from a massive *E. coli* outbreak. Why? Can it simply be explained by saying that some have stronger immune systems than others? In some outbreaks, those with immune systems that are typically strong to certain illnesses such as colds or influenza may still get sick from *E. coli* infections. What is the decisive factor?

The decisive factor is the population and composition of the body's probiotic colonies. The quantity and content of our probiotic populations make the difference between those who are easily sickened and overwhelmed by viral, bacterial or fungal infections.

Illustrating this, *Lactobacillus rhamnosus* GG or a placebo was given to 235 children hospitalized with persistent diarrhea in a randomized, double-blind and controlled study in India (Basu *et al.* 2007). *Escherichia coli* were the most common bacteria infecting the children, followed by *Shigella* spp. and *Clostridium difficile*. The average illness duration was significantly lower among the probiotic group (5.3 days versus 9.2 days), and the average hospital stay was also significantly less among the probiotic group.

Therapeutic Probiotics

Like a planet, the human body houses huge populations of conscious life forms. There are somewhere in the neighborhood of ten times more probiotic bacteria in our bodies than cells. Think about this. This means our bodies are more microbial than cellular. Friendly bacteria make up approximately 70% of our immune system. Scientists are now even suggesting that the DNA of probiotic bacteria is more important than our cells' DNA in predicting our vulnerabilities and possible future diseases.

About one hundred trillion bacteria live in the body's digestive system—about 3.5 pounds worth. The digestive tract contains about 400-500 different bacteria species. About twenty species make up about 75% of the population, however. Many of these are our resident strains, which attach to our intestinal walls. Many others are transient. These transient strains will typically stay for no more than about two weeks.

The majority of our probiotics live in the colon, although billions also live in the mouth and small intestines. Other populations of bacteria and yeast can also live within joints, under the armpits, under the toenails, in the vagina; between the toes; and among the body's various other nooks and body cavities.

Microorganisms living within our bodies may be either *pro*biotic, *patho*biotic or *eu*biotic. A probiotic is a microorganism living within the body while contributing positively to the body's health. These friendly bacteria also are also called intestinal *flora*—meaning "healthful." The pathobiotic is a microorganism that harms or impedes the body in one way or another. Eubiotics can be either harmful or helpful to the body, depending upon their colony size and location. A healthy body contains a substantially greater number of probiotics than pathobiotics, while a diseased body likely contains more pathobiotic than probiotic populations.

Probiotic Inoculation

Our first major encounter with large populations of bacteria comes when our baby body descends the cervix and emerges from the vagina. During this birthing journey—assuming a healthy mother—we are exposed to numerous species of future resident probiotics. This first inoculation provides an advanced immune shield to keep populations of pathobiotics at bay. The inoculation process does not end here, however.

Because we get much of our bacteria as we pass through the vagina, Caesarean section babies have significantly lower colonies of healthy bacteria. *Bifidobacterium infantis* is considered the healthiest probiotic colonizing infants. Some research has indicated that while 60% of vagina-birth babies have *B. infantis* colonies, only 9% of C-section babies are colonized with probiotics, and only 9% of those are colonized with *B. infantis*. This means that less than one percent of C-section babies are properly colonized with *B. infantis*, while 60% of vagina births are colonized with *B. infantis*.

Our body establishes its resident strains during the first year to eighteen months. Following the inoculation from the vagina, these are accomplished from a combination of breast-feeding and putting everything in our mouth, from our parent's fingers to anything we find as we are crawling around the ground. These activities can provide a host of different bacteria—both pathobiotic and probiotic.

Mother's colostrum (early milk) may contain up to 40% probiotics. This will be abundant in bifidobacteria, assuming the mother is not taking antibiotics. Healthy strains of bifidobacteria typically colonize our body first and set up an environment for other groups of bacteria, such as lactobacilli, to more easily become established.

Picking up a good mix of cooperative probiotic species is a crucial part of the establishment of our body's immune system. Some of the probiotic strains we ingest as infants may become permanent residents. They will continue to line the digestive tract to protect against infection while learning to collaborate with our immune system.

Housing the Resident Strains

As these early probiotics set up shop within our intestines and other cavities, they become recognized by the body and incubated in parts of the body's lymphatic system. The vermiform appendix, for example, was observed in 2007 by scientists at Duke University (Randal, *et al.*) as housing resident probiotic strains, and releasing them into the cecum during increased infection. It seems that finally the purpose for the mysterious appendix has been discovered after decades of surgical removal. Other lymph ducts like the tonsils are also suspected to incubate resident probiotic strains as well.

Gaining early probiotic strains from the environment may appear difficult to understand, as we have been taught that dirt is infectious. Rather, natural soils contain huge populations of various bacteria. Many of these are spore-forming *soil-based organisms*. Some soil-based organisms or SBOs can become probiotic populations after early ingestion. Others, which may be less healthy to the body, will allow exposure to probiotic colonies and the immune system to counteract those strains in the future. This training mechanism is critical to the body's future immunity. This means those important infantile occupations— crawling on all fours, eating dirt, making mud pies, having food fights, playing tag and so on—all come together to deliver a stronger immune system later in life.

This has been confirmed by recent research illustrating that infants raised in sterile environments are more likely to suffer from allergies, infections and food sensitivities. Parents should consider living in a natural setting or at least outings to natural environments like pesticide free parks to provide exposure to pathogens and future probiotic colonies.

We can house many transient probiotics, but our resident probiotic bacteria strains do not change through adulthood. Once they take up residence, those strains become part of our body's ecosystem. This does not mean they always remain in strong numbers. Over years of stress, antibiotics and toxin exposure, resident strains may become dramatically reduced.

Supplemented probiotics do not appear to replace these resident strains. Supplemented probiotics typically remain for a couple of weeks, more or less, depending upon the strain and our internal environment. It is believed by some experts that with continued dosing of supplemental strains, resident strains —if they are still present—may regrow in colony strength.

Illustrating strain-specific survival among children, Polish scientists (Szymański *et al.* 2006) gave *Lactobacillus rhamnosus* to children with diarrhea. The researchers found that some *L. rhamnosus* strains given were found among 80% of patients after 5 days, and among 41.3% after 14 days. One particular strain, *L. rhamnosus* 573L/1, "colonized the G.I. tract more persistently," according to the researchers.

Probiotic Gatekeepers

As mentioned, probiotics line mucosal linings around our oral cavity, gums, teeth, nasal cavity, throat, esophagus, and associated membranes. These probiotics deter the entry of pathogenic bacteria, viruses and fungi through the mouth and nose. Assuming the colonies are strong enough, even if the immune system is not able to properly identify or attack the invader, the oral probiotic system will remove the invader in short order. This will be accomplished by the probiotics producing certain acids and antibiotics that either specifically kill that type of invader or create an environment within which the invader does not feel comfortable.

Oral probiotics, for example, will vigorously defend the areas around the gums and teeth. The problem arises when our diets become overly sugary. As we will discuss later in more detail, probiotics require complex oligosaccharides like inulin, FOS (fructooligosaccharides) and GOS (galactooligosaccharides) for food sources. They do not thrive from simple sugars like glucose and sucrose. Pathogenic bacteria, on the other hand, typically thrive from these simple sugars. In fact, they can grow quite quickly, and may immediately begin to outnumber the probiotic populations, causing caries and gum infections.

Within the intestines, probiotics attach to and dwell in between the villi and microvilli. This allows them to not only keep pathogenic bacteria from infecting those cells: It also allows them to monitor food molecule size of nutrients being presented to the intestinal wall for absorption. This helps prevent the body from absorbing molecules that are too large or not sufficiently broken down. As we will discuss further, large, atypical molecules that have entered the bloodstream will stimulate an inflammatory and allergic response. This is because these larger molecules are not recognized by the immune system.

This is often the case with wheat proteins, milk proteins and nut proteins. For many people, they will be able to drink milk or eat nuts or breads for many years. Then suddenly they become allergic or sensitive to the food. Why? Larger proteins from these foods are being allowed into the bloodstream.

The relationship between what is often called intestinal permeability and allergies has been confirmed by a number of studies. We will review a few of these, as well as studies confirming that probiotics can reverse the problem—effectively reducing allergies and intestinal permeability.

The mouth and intestines are not the only places probiotics guard against invaders. The vagina, urinary tract and anus are also inhabited by species of probiotics that guard against microbial intrusion. Healthy colonies of these species protect us against the intrusion of pathogens and toxins into these areas.

Territorial Colonization

Some of our bacteria live peacefully together. Most struggle with other colonies, and mark clearly defined territories with special biochemical secretions. Probiotics within the same colony usually specialize in particular functions. Some work together to help break down foods, and some guard and protect their territory as they consume metabolites. To protect against pathogens, many will produce a number of natural antibiotics designed to reduce the populations of competitors. At the same time, some of their antibiotic secretions aid the body's immune system by stimulating T-cell and B-cell activity.

Many will release antibiotic secretions called bacteriocins that selectively reduce the growth of other pathogens, including yeasts and pathobiotics. In other words, their antibiotic secretions—unlike many pharmaceutical antibiotics—can selectively damage certain strains of pathobiotics and not others. Many probiotics also produce lactic acid, acetic acid, hydrogen peroxide, lactoperoxidase, lipopolysaccharides, and a number of other antimicrobial substances. Lactic acid, for example, helps acidify the intestines and prevent harmful bacteria overgrowth.

To give an idea of just how diligent and efficient probiotic bacteria are in producing antimicrobial components, a study at the Department of Microbiology of the Abaseheb Garware College in India (Watve *et al.* 2001) studied the genus *Steptomyces* since the 1970s, and found that it has been producing new antibiotic substances exponentially over the years. They logistically graphed the count of antimicrobial substances produced over the years, and estimated that the genus is capable of producing more than 100,000 different antibiotic compounds!

Because bacteria are living organisms, they are *adaptable*. This means that they will respond to new competition with new antibiotic tools. They will produce different types of biochemicals, and develop different means of attack.

Most bacteria also manufacture waste products. Some of these are toxic and some of them are beneficial. Pathobiotics manufacture substances that increase the risk of disease by raising the body's toxicity level in addition to infecting cells. Various immunological diseases directly or indirectly stem from the waste streams of pathobiotics. Harmful bacteria can overload the liver and lymph systems with toxins. The toxins produced by bacteria are referred to as endotoxins—a technical name for bacteria poop. Bacteria defecate just as any other living organism does. Endotoxins from pathogenic bacteria can contribute to or directly stimulate inflammation and irritation within the intestines, promoting irritable bowel or colitis, Crohn's, polyps, diverticulitis and/or pouchitis. In comparison, probiotic waste is either healthy or inconsequential to the intestines. In other words, probiotic poop can be good for us!

Finnish scientists (Isolauri *et al.* 1994) gave lactobacilli probiotics to 42 children with acute rotavirus diarrhea. They found that the probiotics significantly reduced levels of the endotoxin urease, and lessened infection duration among the probiotic group compared to the placebo group.

Researchers at the University of Bologna in Italy (Gionchetti *et al.* 2003) reported a study of probiotic administration among patients suffering from Crohn's disease, ulcerative colitis and pouchitis. The study focused on patients that had recently undergone an ileostomy closure. A blend of eight lactobacilli and bifidobacteria or a placebo was given to 40 patients. Of the 20 patients given probiotics, only 10% experienced an acute pouchitis episode versus 40% of the 20 patients given a placebo. This statistically significant difference indicates the important role that probiotic bacteria play, and their ability to reduce intestinal inflammatory diseases.

Most bacteria in the digestive tract are anaerobic. This means they live without the need for oxygen. They can thus live in the darkest, bleakest regions of our bodies—including areas with little circulation. Not all biotics are anaerobic however—some are aerobic and some can go either way. These species will live in regions where they can more easily obtain oxygen—including the mouth, the stomach and the vagina. We might compare this to some species on the earth walking on the land and breathing oxygen, while others—like plants—utilize carbon dioxide.

Friendly Flora Nutrition

Probiotics are also called 'friendly' because they help us digest food and they secrete beneficial nutritional products. Unbelievably, probiotics are a good source of a number of essential nutrients. They can manufacture biotin, thiamin (B1), riboflavin (B2), niacin (B3), pantothenic acid (B5), pyridoxine (B6), cobalamine (B12), folic acid, vitamin A and vitamin K. Their lactic acid secretions also increase the assimilation of minerals that require acid for absorption, such as copper, iron, magnesium and manganese among many others.

Probiotics are also critical to nutrient absorption. They break away amino acids from complex proteins, and mid-chain fatty acids from complex fats. They help break down bile acids. They help convert polyphenols from plant materials into assimilable biomolecules. They also aid in soluble fiber fermentation, yielding digestible fatty acids and sugars. Among many other nutritive tasks, they also help increase the bioavailability of calcium.

Probiotic Nutrition

Biotin	Produced by probiotics
Thiamin (B1)	Produced by probiotics
Riboflavin (B2)	Produced by probiotics
Niacin (B3)	Produced by probiotics
Pantothenic Acid (B5)	Produced by probiotics
Pyridoxine (B6)	Produced by probiotics
Cobalamine (B12)	Produced by probiotics
Folic Acid (B9)	Produced by probiotics
Vitamin A	Produced by probiotics

Vitamin K	Produced by probiotics
Copper	Probiotics increase bioavailability
Calcium	Probiotics increase bioavailability
Magnesium	Probiotics increase bioavailability
Iron	Probiotics increase bioavailability
Manganese	Probiotics increase bioavailability
Potassium	Probiotics increase bioavailability
Zinc	Probiotics increase bioavailability
Proteins	Probiotics break down for digestibility
Fats	Probiotics break down for digestibility
Carbohydrates	Probiotics break down and process
Sugars	Probiotics break down and process
Milk	Probiotics increase digestibility
Phytonutrients	Probiotics increase digestibility
Cholesterol	Probiotics bind to + reduce blood levels

We should note here that not all probiotics produce the same nutrients. Some, in fact, will consume some nutrients that others manufacture. For example, *Lactobacillus bulgaricus* will produce folic acid in yogurt, and *Lactobacillus acidolpholus* will consume folic acid. At the end of the day, a mixture of probiotics will still have a net increase in nutrients, however. For this reason, most cultured dairy products have significantly higher nutrient contents than the milk or cream they were made with.

Probiotics also assist in peristalsis—the rhythmic motion of the digestive tract—by helping move intestinal contents through the system. They also produce antifungal substances such as acidophillin, bifidin and hydrogen peroxide, which counteract the growth of not-so-friendly yeasts. Probiotic hydrogen peroxide secretions are also oxygenating, providing free radical scavenging. In addition, they can manufacture some essential fatty acids, and are the source of 5-10% of all short-chained fatty acids essential for healthy immune system function.

Probiotics directly and indirectly break down toxins utilizing biochemical secretions and colonizing activities. Nutrients produced by probiotics have been found to have antitumor and anticancer effects within the body. Some probiotics can prevent assimilation of toxins like mercury and other heavy metals. Others will directly bind these toxins or will facilitate their binding to other molecules in order to remove them.

Probiotic nutrients are instrumental in slowing cellular degeneration and the diseases associated with it. Through their nutritive mechanisms, probiotics help normalize serum levels of cholesterol and triglycerides. Some probiotics even help break down and rebuild hormones.

Probiotic nutrients can also increase the productivity of the spleen and thymus—the key organs of the immune system.

Probiotics are necessary components to healthy digestion. Their populations dwell along and within the intestinal mucosal lining, providing a protective barrier to assist in the process of filtering and digesting toxins and other matter prior to these toxins encountering the intestinal wall cells. This mechanism helps maintain the brush barrier cells and keep the mucosal lining of our intestines from damage caused by foreign molecules coming from our foods and their metabolites. Damage to the brush cells of the intestinal lining is the prime cause for a number of irritable bowel disorders.

Illustrating probiotic production of one critical nutrient, Italian researchers (Strozzi and Mogna 2008) gave 23 healthy volunteers *Bifidobacterium adolescentis* DSM 18350, *B. adolescentis* DSM 18352, or *Bifidobacterium pseudocatenulatum* DSM 18353. Stool samples taken before and 48 hours after administration showed a significant increase of bioavailable folic acid from each of the probiotic strains.

Probiotics will also compete with pathogenic organisms for nutrients. Assuming good numbers, this strategy can check pathobiotic growth substantially. Nutrients produced by probiotics will also help stimulate the immune cell production, and normalize their activity during inflammatory circumstances.

Dysbiosis

Dysbiosis is a state where the body has an imbalance between probiotic populations and pathogenic bacteria populations. In other words, the system is being overrun by the pathogenic bacteria and there are not enough probiotics in place to control their populations. When the body is lacking probiotics, or is overgrown with pathobiotic populations, there is typically an intestinal infection of some type. The extent of the infection, of course, depends upon the type of pathogenic bacteria present, and their populations in proportion to probiotic populations.

Many disorders can be traced back to dysbiosis. Some are direct and obvious, and some are not so obvious, and often appear as other disorders. In general, most digestive disorders are either caused by or accompanied by a lack of balanced intestinal probiotic populations. There are several types of dysbiosis.

We can usually detect *putrefaction dysbiosis* from the incidence of slow bowel movement. Symptoms of putrefaction dysbiosis include depression, diarrhea, fatigue, memory loss, numbing of hands and feet, sleep disturbances, joint pain and muscle weakness. Many of these disorders and others are often due directly to the overgrowth of pathobiotics. The bacteria are burdening the blood stream with endotoxin waste products and neurotoxins; infecting cells, joints, nerves, brain tissues and other regions of the body.

Another overgrowth issue is *fermentation dysbiosis.* This is often evidenced by bloating, constipation, diarrhea, fatigue, and gas; and the faulty digestion of carbohydrates, grains, proteins and fiber. This is also a result of pathobiotic overgrowth, but in this type of dysbiosis, yeasts are prevalent among the overgrowth populations. As we know from baking bread, yeast will ferment quickly in warm, humid environments.

Either type of dysbiosis can result in an acute case of watery diarrhea. While diarrhea in itself may not sound that dangerous, the critical loss of body water will result in dehydration, which can be lethal. This is because the body's water is being purged faster than our ability to replace it.

A few years ago, researchers (Allen *et al.* 2004) published a review of twenty-three studies that trialed probiotics on patients with acute diarrhea. These twenty-three studies were randomized and controlled, and carefully chosen to meet stringent control criteria. Together the review gathered data on 1,917 patients in countries with low infant mortality rates. The overall conclusion of this review was that probiotics reduced the risk of infection substantially, and the duration of diarrhea episodes by an average of 30.48 hours.

For example, German scientists (Rosenfeldt, *et al.* 2002) gave sixty-nine children hospitalized with rotavirus enteritis a placebo or the probiotics *Lactobacillus rhamnosus* or *Lactobacillus reuteri* twice per day for five days. The probiotic treatment group had a significantly reduced period of rotavirus excretion, reduced hospital stays and duration of episodes. Studying another group of forty-three children with mild gastroenteritis recruited from day care centers, the researchers found that probiotic treatment resulted in average diarrhea episode lengths of 76 hours—versus 116 hours among the non-probiotic group.

A body with low probiotic populations will create havoc for the immune system. *Deficiency dysbiosis* is related to an absence of probiotics, leading to damaged intestinal mucosa. This can lead to irritable bowel syndrome, food sensitivities, and intestinal permeability. The lack of probiotics allows the intestinal wall to come into contact with foreign molecules. This can open up the junctions between the intestinal brush barrier cells. This can in turn lead to the entry of these toxins along with larger more complex food particles into the bloodstream—such as larger peptides and protein molecules—as we have discussed. Because these molecules are not normally found in the blood stream, the immune system identifies them as foreigners. The body then launches an inflammatory immune response, leading to *sensitization dysbiosis*. Linked to probiotic deficiency, sensitization dysbiosis causes food intolerances, food allergies, chemical and food sensitivities, acne, connective tissue disease and psoriasis. Intestinal permeability has also been suspected in a variety of lung and joint infections.

Research has directly connected dysbiosis and intestinal probiotics with nasal and lung infections. Illustrating this, Swiss scientists (Glück and Gebbers 2003) recruited 209 healthy adults. Upon examination, many were found to have nasal-cavity inhabitation of either *Staphylococcus aureus*, *Streptococcus pneumoniae* or *b-hemolytic Streptococci*—all potentially dangerous pathogens. One hundred and eight of these adults consumed a probiotic beverage containing *L. rhamnosus* GG, *L. acidophilus* 145, *S. thermophilus* and *Bifidobacterium* sp. B420 each day for three weeks. The rest consumed standard yogurt containing only *S. thermophilus* and *L. bulgaricus* at lower dosages per day. After three weeks, exams of all subjects showed that infection rates among the probiotic group dropped 19% while little or no change occurred in the control group.

The obvious signs of dysbiosis include hormonal imbalances and mood swings, high cholesterol, vitamin B deficiencies, frequent gas and bloating, indigestion, irritable bowels, easy bruising of the skin, constipation, diarrhea, vaginal infections, reduced sex drive, prostate enlargement, food sensitivities, chemical sensitivities, bladder infections, allergies, rhinovirus and rotavirus infections, influenza, and various histamine-related inflammatory syndromes such as rashes, asthma and skin irritation.

Illustrating the connection between probiotics and skin irritations, Denmark children 1-13 years of age diagnosed with atopic dermatitis were tested in a double blind, placebo-controlled crossover study (Rosenfeldt *et al.* 2003). Freeze-dried *L. rhaminosus* 19070-2 and *L. reuteri* DSM 122460 probiotics were administered for six weeks. The children were then examined for symptoms, and 56% reported improved eczema compared to 15% among the control group.

Furthermore, the infection of various parts of the body—either from pathogenic bacteria or their endotoxins—can cause various ailments typically associated with autoimmune or degenerative etiologies. Autoimmune type diseases of the liver, the urinary tract, the joints, gums and ears, heart and lungs can directly result from any one of the above forms of dysbiosis. An example of this is Grave's disease—considered a classic autoimmune disorder caused seemingly by the immune system attacking healthy cells of the thyroid gland. Tests have shown that some 80% of Grave's sufferers test positive for *Yersinia enterocolitica* antibodies. Dysbiosis is often accompanied by an overgrowth of the bacteria, *Yersinia enterocolitica.* Yersina endotoxins can attach to thyroid cells, stimulating the over-production of thyroid hormone—one of the symptoms of Grave's disease.

The Progression of Dysbiosis

When pathogenic bacteria take over and begin to control the digestive tract, a variety of symptoms will develop. This is because pathogenic bacteria produce toxins that can alter the health of the intestinal wall cells, and leak into the bloodstream, where they can damage and burden the immune system. Over time, these toxins begin to alter the make up and efficiency of the cells they come into contact with. Cells can also become directly infected by bacteria.

These toxic substances begin to change the way many cells operate. This precipitates a change in the genetic expression of those cells. When a cell must adapt to a toxic environment, its epigenetic DNA expression will eventually mirror this adjustment. This mutation subtly changes the identity and activity of the cell, which stimulates the immune system's inflammatory response to rid the body of the mutated cells. This pattern is apparent in autoimmune diseases including Crohn's disease, irritable bowel syndrome, allergies, arthritis, fibromyalgia, interstitial cystitis and many other autoimmune disorders. While it may be difficult to directly connect the loss of the body's probiotic colonies with these diseases, as we will discover, their absence allows pathogenic bacteria to grow and increasingly burden the body and immune system with endotoxins.

As dysbiosis progresses, it can play a dramatic role in the incidence of food sensitivities and food allergies. Without probiotic colonies positioned along the intestinal wall, large food particles can become absorbed into the bloodstream. Once absorbed, these larger-than-normal molecules are subject to attack by the body's immune response. During this inflammatory response, histamines are generated, which cause the sinus cavities to explode with sneezing and watering of the eyes.

The further progression of dysbiosis can result in the microbial or endotoxin invasion of remote tissue systems around the body. Should the protective layer of probiotic colonies along the intestinal wall become diminished, pathobiotic spores and endotoxins can escape into the bloodstream. Once they land in protective tissue systems, the spores can grow into colonies, releasing bacteria that can infect and damage surrounding systems, including the heart, the liver, the kidneys and even the joints. Even in locations pathobiotics can't reach, their endotoxins can damage these remote cells and tissue systems.

For example, increasingly, medical research is demonstrating that some arthritic conditions are attributed directly to infectious bacteria. Spores, endotoxins and even grown bacteria have been found within synovial tissues and fluids. How did they get there? The progression of dysbiosis is the smoking gun. Once pathobiotics accumulate in the joints they will multiply, because joints provide some protection from the circulating immune system. Once identified by the body's defense systems, the body launches an inflammatory attack, resulting in the swelling and pain associated with septic and rheumatoid arthritis.

A number of reputable health experts have concluded that a variety of other internal diseases may result from or be related to the various forms of dysbiosis. Strong results from the research are also supporting this conclusion, as we will discuss in depth in the next chapter. We will also show how probiotics have the ability to protect against tumor development and prevent or improve the prognosis of a variety of ailments.

Probiotics and Disease

The medicinal use of cultured and fermented foods dates back thousands of years. Probiotics have been used by the Egyptian, Roman, Greek, Asian, Northern Europe and Eastern European civilizations. These ancient societies found that probiotic cultures not only could preserve foods: They also provided many health benefits.

About a century ago, Nobel laureate and Russian professor Ilya Metchnikov proposed the idea to western medicine that these healthy benefits were derived from tiny probiotic microorganisms.

Science is still unfolding the complex mechanisms and many benefits derived from the more than 500 species of still largely unresearched microorganisms that inhabit our bodies from head to toe with vast populations concentrated in our intestinal tracts.

"Death begins in the colon," Metchnikov is reported to have said. Metchnikov is most recognized in western science for the discovery of phagotosis by white blood cells. He became focused upon probiotics after noticing that some Eastern European villagers from Bulgaria and Serbia who ate yogurt were living longer—some beyond 100 years of age. Through the process of elimination, it seemed that the yogurt was the consistent variable between those that remained healthy among these societies—during a period where many in Europe and Russia were expiring in their 40s and 50s.

Western science's fifty-year experiment with prescriptive antibiotic use is showing signs of failure. Infectious disease rates are rising. Pathogenic bacteria have devised "superbug" facilities to outmaneuver our static antibiotics.

Thankfully, this is escorting in a new era of research. Medical researchers are realizing, as Metchnikov did, that probiotics may provide the solution for a number of disease pathologies.

Early research on probiotics focused upon intestinal infections. Then researchers began cruelly testing probiotics on animals—submitting them to inflicted infections or diseases like cancer and treating them with probiotics. Some astounding results came out of this research. This research was not ready to be embraced by the medical community, however. In addition, supplemental probiotics were plagued with quality and dosage problems, because few understood how to properly produce and package them. This led to inconsistent results, both among human clinical research and use by the general population.

The combination of these problems produced a backlash of negative reviews about probiotics several decades ago—one that is still to some degree plaguing research results.

Over time, however, enough successes among *in vitro* and *in vivo* studies have brought more investment and focus into probiotic research. This has opened the doors for human clinical research—which has established increasingly clear evidence on the effectiveness of probiotics for a number of ailments.

Here we will review a sampling of research in a number of human disease pathologies. We should mention that there have also been some clinical studies that have shown little effectiveness among some of these same diseases. Explaining these inconsistencies is quite easy, however. Probiotics are living organisms. They can be produced in a variety of mediums and environments. They can also be extracted from those mediums differently and packaged within different products. In addition, each species and strain may respond differently to each type of culture medium and packaging. Some cultures can easily die, as periodic studies on supplemental viability have confirmed.

Some of the probiotic studies have utilized dairy mediums and traditional yogurt making to culture the probiotics used. Others used extracted freeze-dried probiotics. Still others used heat-killed bacteria, believing that the dead bacteria would have the same effects. It is true that because probiotics produce antibiotics within their culture medium, the medium after the bacteria are dead can be effective for some ailments. This, of course, is the same general strategy used to make pharmaceutical antibiotics. While some of these heat-killed probiotic studies showed success, many showed little or no effects compared to the living bacteria studies. As we have discussed, living bacteria adjust their strategies and antibiotics to different types of pathogens.

Noting the variance of probiotic cultures used for much of the research, the possibility is quite large that many of the studies that showed little or no effectiveness were utilizing probiotics that were dead upon arrival: They could have been killed by heat, light, centrifuging, processing, storage or packaging. They could have also been killed by the acids in the stomach. It is quite easy, as we'll discuss, to kill off entire populations of probiotics. They are quite sensitive creatures and need to be handled carefully.

In summary, this lack of standardization among probiotic culturing and handling certainly does not bode well for consistent results, and easily explains why some probiotic studies have shown tremendously positive results, while others have not shown the same effects.

The bottom line is that those studies that have showed positive results are clear evidence for the incredible effects of these tiny warriors. They also indicate the need for further standardization and further research.

Whether mentioned or not, almost every one of the studies in the following sections were randomized, placebo-controlled and double-blinded or blinded studies. While the strain numbers have been left in, this is not a statement that only that strain of that species will have that particular effect. While it has been shown in some studies that different strains of the same species can have different effects, this has not been proven conclusively to be true in all cases, as we'll discuss further in detail.

Rotavirus and Intestinal Bacterial Infections

Intestinal infections leading to acute diarrhea are often caused by an overgrowth of certain bacteria or fungi within the intestines. This has been the most researched clinical use of probiotics, particularly among children, where diarrhea can easily cause death. Here is a sampling of the hundreds of clinical research on probiotics and intestinal infections:

Researchers from the Department of Pediatrics at Italy's University of Naples Federico II (Canani *et al.* 2007) investigated five different probiotics for the treatment of acute diarrhea among children. 571 children diagnosed with acute diarrhea received either 1) a placebo; 2) *Lactobacillus rhamnosus* strain GG; *Saccharomyces boulardii;* 3) *Bacillus clausii;* 4) *Enterococcus faecium* SF68; 5) or a combination of *L delbrueckii* var *bulgaricus, Streptococcus thermophilus, Lactobacillus acidophilus,* and *Bifidobacterium bifidum.* The average illness duration was significantly less for the probiotic group who took the combination of four strains (at 70 hours) and *L. rhamnosus* (at 78.5 hours), as compared with the placebo group (at 115.0 hours). The other probiotics given were not significantly better than the placebo.

Scientists from the University College of Medical Sciences and GTB Hospital in India (Agarwal and Bhasin 2002) studied 150 children with acute diarrhea. The children were given fermented milk with 1) a combination of *Lactobacillus casei* DN-114001, *Lactobacillus bulgaricus* and *Streptococcus thermophilus;* 2) Indian dahl supplemented with *Lactococcus lactis, Lactococcus lactis cremoris* and *Leuconostac mesenteroide;* 3) or a heat-treated yogurt with no live bacteria. Both live probiotic groups showed a significant reduction of illness compared to the heat-treated yogurt. The greatest reduction occurred with the *Lactobacillus casei* fermented milk.

Researchers from the Faculty of Medicine at London's Imperial College (Hickson *et al.* 2007) studied 135 elderly patients infected with *Clostridium difficile.* They were given a placebo or a combination of *Lactobacillus casei, Lactobacillus bulgaricus,* and *Streptococcus thermophilus* while taking antibiotics and then for one additional week after the antibiotic treatment was completed. Twelve percent of the probiotic group developed diarrhea (related to antibiotics) compared to 34% among the placebo group.

Italian scientists (Guarino *et al.* 1997) gave 100 children with rotavirus and non-rotavirus diarrhea a placebo or the probiotic *Lactobacillus rhamnosus* GG (also referred to as *Lactobacillus* GG). The duration of diarrhea was reduced from 6 to 3 days in all children (both rotavirus and non-rotavirus) receiving *Lactobacillus* GG.

Swedish researchers gave 26 adult volunteers with clostridia intestinal infections either a placebo or *Lactobacillus plantarum* DSM 9843. After 3 weeks, the probiotic group had significantly less sulfite-reducing clostridia (Johansson *et al.* 1998).

Scientists from the Liverpool School of Tropical Medicine (Raza *et al.* 1995) gave probiotics or placebo to 40 children hospitalized with acute diarrhea in Pakistan. Averaging 13 months of age, the children were given either *Lactobacillus* GG or the placebo for 2 days. The number of children with persistent watery diarrhea at 48 hours was 31% in the probiotic group versus 75% in the placebo group.

Researchers from the Universidad de Buenos Aires' Medical School (Gaón *et al.* 2003) tested 89 children aged 6-24 months with persistent diarrhea. They received a placebo, a combination of *Lactobacillus casei* and *Lactobacillus acidophilus,* or *Saccharomyces boulardii* for five days. Both probiotic treatments were effective in significantly improving those children compared to the placebo.

Scientists from Argentina's Universidad de Buenos Aires (Gaon *et al.* 2002) also studied 22 patients with chronic diarrhea. They were given either *Lactobacillus casei* and *Lactobacillus acidophilus* or placebo for three periods of seven days with untreated periods in between. The probiotic combination significantly reduced the diarrhea compared to the placebo group. In addition, probiotic effects were significantly reduced during the untreated periods, leading the researchers to suggest that continual use provides better efficacy.

Researchers from the Cathay General Hospital's Department of Pediatrics (Lee *et al.* 2001) studied one hundred hospitalized children with acute diarrhea. They were given either *Lactobacillus acidophilus* and *Bifidobacterium infantis* or a placebo for four days. The diarrhea frequency among the probiotic group improved on the first and second day of hospitalization significantly more than the placebo group.

In a multicenter study from France's Centre Hospitalier Universitaire de Grenoble (Chouraqui *et al.* 2004), *Bifidobacterium lactis* or placebo was given in formula to 90 healthy children for 8 months living in residential nurseries or foster care centers. The probiotic group had a 28.3% incidence of diarrhea compared to 38.7% among the placebo group. As for episode duration, the probiotic group had an average of 1.15 days of diarrhea compared to 2.3 days in the control group.

Scientists from Italy's University of degli Studi Pediatric Department (Michielutti *et al.* 1996) studied 63 children under 4 years old infected with intestinal bacteria. They were divided into three groups. One group was given *Lactobacillus acidophilus*. The other was given a placebo. The third group was given both antibiotic therapy and *L. acidophilus*. The first (probiotic-only) group showed significant clinical improvement over the second group. The third group illustrated that the probiotic therapy mitigated the adverse effects of dysbiosis following antibiotic treatment.

Finnish scientists from the University of Tampere (Kaila *et al.* 1995) tested the difference of effects between live and heat inactivated *Lactobacillus* GG on the immune system in patients with rotavirus infections. Their results in a rotavirus serum IgA enzyme immunoassay showed that antibody responses were significantly greater among infants treated with live *Lactobacillus* GG. While 10 of 12 infants receiving the live probiotics showed rotavirus-specific IgA secreting cells, only 2 of 13 infants receiving inactivated (dead) *Lactobacillus* GG showed the IgA secreting cells.

This is not to say that even dead probiotics do not lessen intestinal infections. Seventy-three children with diarrhea—50% of whom had rotavirus—were given either heat-killed *L. acidophilus* LB or a placebo. In 24 hours after treatment, the probiotic group had significantly less diarrhea. At the end of the study, the probiotics group had diarrhea for an average of 43 hours and the placebo group had diarrhea for an average of 57 hours (Simakachorn *et al.* 2000).

Scientists from Ramathibodi Hospital in Bangkok (Phuapradit *et al.* 1999) gave 175 children aged from 6 to 36 months old a placebo, *Bifidobacterium* Bb12 alone, or *Bifidobacterium* Bb12 combined with *Streptococcus thermophilus* in formula. During the 8-month study period, the non-probiotic group had a 4-fold increase in the IgA antibody titer for rotavirus, while both the *Bifidobacterium* Bb12 alone group and the group treated with Bb12 combined with *Streptococcus thermophilus* had no significant changes in their IgA antibody titer throughout the study period. This led the researchers to conclude that, "children receiving bifidobacteria-supplemented milk-based formula may be protected against symptomatic rotavirus infection."

Researchers from the Johns Hopkins University School of Medicine (Saavedra *et al.* 1994) gave *Bifidobacterium bifidum* and *Streptococcus thermophilus* or placebo to infants aged from 5 to 24 months old in a double-blind, placebo-controlled study. In all, 55 infants were assessed for 4,447 patient-days over a 17-month period. During the test period, 31% of the placebo infants developed diarrhea versus 7% of the probiotic group. In addition, 39% of the placebo group shed rotavirus during the study period versus 10% of the probiotic group.

Lactobacillus acidophilus and *Bifidobacterium infantis* probiotics were given to 1,237 newborns placed in intensive care at the Childrens University Hospital Lorencita Villegas in Bogotá, Colombia over one year (Hoyos 1999). The results were compared to (controls) 1,282 newborns not given probiotics while being hospitalized during the previous year. In the previous year, the controls experienced 85 cases of necrotizing enterocolitis, compared to 34 cases among the probiotic newborns. Furthermore, there were 35 NEC-associated deaths among the 1,282 newborns the previous year and only 14 fatalities among the 1,237 newborns given probiotics.

In research from two Finnish hospitals (Shornikova *et al.* 1997), 66 children between six months and three years of age with rotavirus infections and watery diarrhea were given a placebo or two dosages of *Lactobacillus reuteri* for up to 5 days. By the second day, watery diarrhea continued among 80% of the placebo group. In comparison, watery diarrhea continued among only 48% of the large dosage *L. reuteri* group.

Researchers at Spain's Hospital Materno-Infantil Vall d'Hebron (Tormo *et al.* 2006) treated 35 infants with gastrointestinal problems with either standard milk (placebo) or milk fermented milk *Lactobacillus casei* and *Streptococcus thermophilus*. The probiotic milk group was given the probiotic for six weeks and the placebo for six weeks. The placebo group drank the standard milk for twelve weeks. After the testing period, those receiving the probiotics showed a significant reduction of gastrointestinal gram-negative bacteria and an increase in secretory IgA levels (from 2.5 mg/dl to 3.4 mg/dl). Stool exams also confirmed the survival of *L. casei* through the gastrointestinal tract.

Cholesterol

One of the most important indicators of heart or cardiovascular disease is atherosclerosis—the hardening and thickening of the arteries. Atherosclerosis occurs as artery walls are damaged from oxidized low-density lipoproteins, initiating an inflammatory response. Lipoproteins transport cholesterol and triglycerides through the bloodstream as either very-low density (VLDL), low-density (LDL), intermediate-density or high-density lipoproteins (HDL).

Cholesterol comes from our diet and from liver synthesis—which is sent with bile into the intestines. Here it is absorbed into the blood through the intestinal wall and transported via lipoproteins. Higher VLDL-c and LDL-c levels tend to oxidize more quickly, so these tend to cause more artery inflammation. HDL-cholesterol, on the other hand, does not oxidize as easily.

Probiotics will bind to and prevent LDL-cholesterol from being released back into the bloodstream. This effect reduces levels of cholesterol, and more importantly, levels of LDL-cholesterol in the blood. By reducing LDL-c and increasing HDL-c, less oxidation will take place and less artery damage will result.

Scientists from Denmark's The Royal Veterinary and Agricultural University (Agerholm-Larsen *et al.* 2000) gave 70 overweight and obese adult volunteers 1) placebo pills; 2) a placebo yogurt; 3) a yogurt with two strains of *Streptococcus thermophilus* and two strains of *Lactobacillus acidophilus*; 4) a yogurt with two strains of *Streptococcus thermophilus* and one strain of *Lactobacillus rhamnosus*; or 5) a yogurt with one strain of *Enterococcus faecium* and two strains of *Streptococcus thermophilus*. After eight weeks, LDL-cholesterol decreased by 8.4% (0.26) while fibrinogen increased (0.74) in the *Enterococcus faecium-Streptococcus thermophilus* group (#4). Groups #3 and #4 showed significant decreases in blood pressure as well.

Twenty healthy men were given either milk fermented with *Lactobacillus casei* or a placebo for eight weeks in a double-blind, placebo-controlled study from Japan (Kawase *et al.* 2000). Blood samples were taken before, after 4 weeks and after 8 weeks. After 4 and 8 weeks, the high-density lipoprotein cholesterol levels (HDL-c) were significantly higher for the probiotic group while the placebo group showed no change. The probiotic group also had lower triglycerides levels after 4 weeks while the placebo group showed no change.

Scientists from the University of Kentucky (Anderson and Gilliland 1999) conducted two studies: One a single-blind study, and the other a double-blind, placebo-controlled, crossover study. Volunteers completed three and four week trials with either placebo or two different strains of *L. acidophilus*. The combined analysis of both probiotic studies showed a 2.9% reduction in serum cholesterol. The authors commented that this converts to a potential 6 to 10% lowering of coronary heart disease.

Researchers from the Tehran University of Medical Sciences (Ataie-Jafari *et al.* 2009) gave 14 healthy subjects with serum total cholesterol levels of 200 to 300 mg/dL 300 grams of ordinary yogurt or yogurt fermented with *Lactobacillus acidophilus* and *Bifidobacterium lactis*. After the six-week period, the probiotic yogurt group showed a significant decrease in total cholesterol levels compared to the ordinary yogurt group.

Forty-three volunteers were given either a placebo or *Enterococcus faecium* M-74 plus 50 micrograms of organically bound selenium in a double-blind, placebo-controlled study (Hlivak *et al.* 2005). After 56 weeks, total cholesterol among the probiotic group reduced from 229 to 201 mg/dL. LDL cholesterol fell from 149 to 119 mg/dL. No significant changes were seen in the placebo group. The researchers concluded that *E. faecium* reduced serum cholesterol by 12% during the test period.

Researchers from Germany's Friedrich Schiller University (Kiessling *et al.* 2002) first gave 300 grams of control yogurt (with starter culture of *Streptococcus thermophilus* and *Lactobacillus lactis*) per day to 29 women for seven weeks. Then they had 18 women eat the same amount of yogurt enhanced with *Lactobacillus acidophilus* 145 and *Bifidobacterium longum* 913 per day while the others ate the control yogurt for the next seven weeks. During the third seven weeks, the two groups from the second period were reversed. After testing with all groups, the probiotic-enhanced groups had an average of 11.6 mg/dL increase in HDL cholesterol. Levels of LDL and total cholesterol were unchanged.

Scientists from The Netherlands' Nutrition and Food Research Institute in Zeist (Schaafsma *et al.* 1998) gave 32 healthy men either a placebo milk or milk fermented with yogurt starter, *Lactobacillus acidophilus* and fructooligosaccharides. After two treatment periods of three weeks separated by a week off, the probiotic group had 4.4% less total cholesterol and 5.4% lower LDL-cholesterol.

Japanese researchers (Xiao *et al.* 2003) gave yogurt with a combination of *Streptococcus thermophilus* and *Lactobacillus delbrueckii* subsp. bulgaricus (SL), or the same combination with *Bifidobacterium longum* strain BL1 to 32 human subjects with total cholesterol from 220 to 280 mg/dL. After four weeks, the total cholesterol reduced by half in the *B. longum* group, while the cholesterol levels among the normal yogurt group remained nearly unchanged.

In research from Germany's Friedrich Schiller University (Klein *et al.* 2008), 26 healthy volunteers took a yogurt supplement with probiotic strains *L. acidophilus* 74-2 and *B. lactis* 420 or a placebo for five weeks. After the five weeks, they were tested and crossed over. Final test results revealed that the probiotic group's triglyceride levels decreased by 11.6%. Immune system granulocytes and monocytes with phagocytic activity significantly increased in the probiotic group as well.

Blood Pressure

We might wonder how bacteria can lower blood pressure. Blood pressure is increased through an enzyme called ACE (angiotensin-converting enzyme). The ACE pathway, however, can be inhibited by two different tripeptides: isoleucyl-prolyl-proline (IPP) and valyl-prolyl-proline (VPP). These two tripeptides have been found in sour milks fermented with probiotic bacteria. Additional research (Narva *et al.* 2004) has indicated that probiotic-fermented dairy stimulate higher calcium levels than unfermented dairy. Higher serum calcium has also been associated with reduced blood pressure—and lower levels of osteoporosis.

Researchers from the University of Helsinki (Jauhiaimen *et al.* 2005) gave *Lactobacillus helveticus* LBK-16H fermented milk or placebo to 94 high blood pressure patients not receiving medications. After 10 weeks and a 4-week open period, the probiotic group had an average 4.1 mm Hg lower systolic and 1.8 mm Hg lower diastolic blood pressure.

Japanese scientists (Aihara *et al.* 2005) gave either *Lactobacillus helveticus* or a placebo to 40 high blood pressure patients for 4 weeks. During the treatment period, the probiotic group's blood pressure trended slightly higher than the placebo group, but at the end of the four weeks, the probiotic group had 5.0 mm Hg less diastolic blood pressure than the placebo group. No other changes, including pulse rate, was observed.

In the *L. casei* study mentioned earlier (Kawase *et al.* 2000), after 4 and 8 weeks, systolic blood pressure lowered significantly among the probiotic group, while there was no change in the placebo group.

This effect was also seen in the Agerholm-Larsen study mentioned earlier. *Enterococcus faecium* and *Streptococcus thermophilus* produced significant decreases in blood pressure in addition to their cholesterol-lowering effects.

Scientists from the Poland's Pomeranian Academy of Medicine (Naruszewicz *et al.* 2002) gave *Lactobacillus plantarum* 299v or placebo to 36 healthy smoker volunteers for six weeks, in a study we discussed earlier. The probiotic group had significant decreases in systolic blood pressure, leptin levels, and fibrinogen levels. No changes were observed among the placebo group.

Researchers from Finland's National Public Health Institute (Tuomilehto *et al.* 2004) gave 60 hypertensive volunteers not taking medication a placebo or *Lactobacillus helveticus* in fermented milk. During the first study period, the probiotic group had a 2 mmHg more reduction in systolic BP than the placebo group. During the second period, the crossover group experienced an average of 2.6 mmHg lower systolic blood pressure and 1.0 mmHg lower diastolic blood pressure.

Scientists from Tokyo's Kyorin University School of Medicine gave *Lactobacillus helveticus* and *Saccharomyces cerevisiae* fermented milk or placebo to 30 elderly high blood pressure patients—many taking antihypertensive medications. After 8 weeks, the probiotic group's systolic blood pressure decreased 14.1 mmHg. The probiotic group's diastolic blood pressure also decreased, by 6.9 mmHg. The placebo group, on the other hand, had no reduction in blood pressure.

Liver Disease

The liver is one of the body's most important organs. It produces hundreds of thousands of enzymes, helps clear and detoxify the blood, and converts various nutrients into useable molecules. In liver disease such as cirrhosis, the cells of the liver become deranged or diseased. This decreases their effectiveness. Should enough of these hepatocytes become damaged, the liver can shut down. The American Liver Foundation estimates that more than 42,000 Americans die from liver disease every year. One in ten of us have some form of liver disease.

Probiotics interact significantly with the liver. Not only do probiotics help digest food: They also protect the liver and signal to the immune system when a threat to the liver exists. It is no coincidence that alcohol—which is tremendously damaging to the liver—also damages our body's probiotics.

Researchers from Russia's Northern State Medical University (Kirpich *et al.* 2008) studied 66 adult Russian males admitted to a psychiatric hospital with a diagnosis of alcoholic psychosis. They gave the patients standard therapy (abstinence plus vitamins) with *Bifidobacterium bifidum* and *Lactobacillus plantarum* 8PA3 or standard therapy alone without probiotics for five days. Stool cultures and liver enzymes were examined and compared with 24 healthy, matched non-drinker controls. The alcoholic patients had significantly fewer bifidobacteria, lactobacilli, and enterococci than did the healthy non-drinkers. The average starting levels of liver enzymes alanine aminotransferase (ALT), aspartate aminotransferase (AST), and gamma-glutamyl transpeptidase (GGT) were significantly greater in the alcoholic group compared to the healthy non-drinkers.

After 5 days of daily probiotics, alcoholic patients had significantly more bifidobacteria and lactobacilli populations compared to the control group. The probiotic group also had significantly lower AST and ALT levels at the end of treatment than the standard therapy control group. Of the 26 patients with mild alcoholic hepatitis, probiotic therapy significantly reduced liver enzymes ALT, AST, GGT, lactate dehydrogenase and total bilirubin. The researchers concluded that, "Short-term oral supplementation with *B. bifidum* and *L. plantarum* 8PA3 was associated with restoration of the bowel flora and greater improvement in alcohol-induced liver injury than standard therapy alone."

Scientists from Italy's University of Catania (Malaguarnera *et al.* 2007) gave 60 cirrhotic patients *Bifidobacterium longum* plus fructo-oligosaccharides (FOS) or placebo. After 90 days, fasting NH(4) serum levels significantly decreased among the probiotic patients. Other liver tests, including MMSE, Trail Making Test-A and Test-B also significantly improved among the probiotic group as compared with the placebo group.

Researchers from the Liver Failure Group and The Institute of Hepatology at the University College London's Medical School (Stadlbauer *et al.* 2008) studied neutrophil function and cytokine responses in alcoholic cirrhosis patients in an open-label study. Twenty patients with alcoholic cirrhosis were treated with a placebo or *Lactobacillus casei* Shirota for 4 weeks. The data were also compared to 13 healthy control subjects who did not receive probiotics. The cirrhosis patients' starting neutrophil phagocytic capacity was significantly lower than healthy controls (73% versus 98%) before probiotic treatment. Neutrophil phagocytic capacities after the probiotic treatments were equal among the cirrhosis patients and healthy volunteers at the end of the study—while the placebo group's neutrophil capacity did not change. In addition, endotoxin-stimulated TNF-receptor-1, TNFR-2 and interleukin IL10 levels were significantly lower among the probiotic group. The researchers concluded that, "Our data provide a proof-of-concept that probiotics restore neutrophil phagocytic capacity in cirrhosis, possibly by changing IL10 secretion and TLR4 expression."

China's Capital University of Medical Sciences and the Beijing Friendship Hospital (Zhao *et al.* 2004) studied fifty patients with liver cirrhosis. They tested and graded the entire group for intestinal probiotic content and severity of liver disease. The researchers found that the cirrhosis was directly associated with intestinal probiotic content. The more severe the cirrhosis, the more imbalanced the intestinal probiotic content was. The patients were randomized and given *Bifidobacterium*, *Lactobacillus acidophilus* and *Enterococcus faecium*; or *Bacillus subtilis* and *Enterococcus faecium* for 14 days. Fecal flora, pH and ammonia content, and plasma endotoxin levels were tested before and after. All levels improved after both probiotic treatments. In addition, those given *B. subtilis* and *E. faecium* showed a reduction in endotoxin levels among endotoxemia cirrhosis cases.

Researchers from the Department of Surgery at Japan's Nagoya University Graduate School of Medicine (Kanazawa *et al.* 2005) investigated the effects of *L. casei* with 54 patients following hepatectomy. Infection complications were 19% in the probiotic group and 52% in the placebo group.

Forty cirrhosis patients with hepatic encephalopathy were studied by researchers from the University of Naples (Loguercio, *et al.* 1987). They were given either *Enterococcus* probiotic strain SF68 or lactulose (standard treatment) for 10 days. The probiotics were as effective as lactulose in lowering blood ammonia and improving mental state. The beneficial effects of the probiotics persisted significantly longer after treatment was discontinued, however. In addition, reports of diarrhea and abdominal pain with lactulose treatment did not occur with probiotic treatment.

Gum Disease and Dental Caries (Cavities)

The gums and teeth are coated with legions of different bacteria—some probiotic and some pathogenic. Typical oral bacteria include *Streptococcus mutans, Streptococcus salivarius, Lactobacillus salivarius, E. coli, Streptococcus pyogenes, Porphyromonas gingivalis, Tannerella forsynthensis* and *Prevotella intermedia*. With a diet containing too many simple sugars and poor dental hygiene, the pathogenic bacteria can overwhelm the probiotics, causing infected gums and teeth. As pathogenic populations of *S. mutans, S. pyogenes, P. gingivalis, T. forsynthensis* and *P. intermedia* come into greater numbers, serious infections can occur. These conditions are often symptomized by gingivitis, teeth root infection, jawbone infections and general periodontal disease.

Streptococcus mutans was first isolated in 1924, but it was not linked to dental caries until the early 1960s. *S. mutans* and other cavity-forming bacteria consume sugars and carbohydrates from our foods, and produce destructive acids. These acids interact with the calcium in our tooth enamel, forming plaque. It is this interaction and plaque-formation that create cavities. There is now reason to believe that, like probiotics, *S. mutans* can be passed on from mother to infant.

This leads us to wonder whether *Streptococcus mutans* might actually be a eubiotic: a probiotic at controlled colony sizes. Like some other eubiotic yeasts and bacteria, perhaps it is a natural resident of the mouth that simply has grown beyond its healthy populations because of our eating and lifestyle imbalances.

All of the bacteria mentioned above and others can reside in both healthy and infected mouths. The strategy promoted by the modern medical and dental industries is to try to kill virtually all bacteria with various antiseptic mouthwashes and toothpastes. As we can see from continuing statistics on gingivitis and dental caries, these strategies are not working very well. A better strategy may be to use nature's probiotic populations to create a balance between the healthy bacteria and the disease-promoting bacteria. If probiotic populations are maximized, they will deplete and manage the pathogenic bacteria populations.

Let's see how this is supported by the research:

Researchers from the Istanbul's Yeditepe University Dental School (Caglar *et al.* 2008) gave oral lozenges of *Lactobacillus reuteri* or placebo to 20 healthy young women. After sucking on one lozenge a day for 10 days, salivary *Streptococcus mutans* levels were significantly reduced among the probiotic group, compared to the placebo group and before treatment.

Scientists from Yeditepe University (Caglar *et al.* 2007) gave placebo or *Lactobacillus reuteri* probiotic chewing gums to 80 healthy young adults for three weeks. The *L. reuteri* gums significantly reduced levels of salivary *Streptococcus mutans* compared to placebo and before treatment.

Scientists from Italy's University of L'Aquila, Department of Experimental Medicine (Riccia *et al.* 2007) gave 8 healthy volunteers and 21 chronic periodontitis patients *Lactobacillus brevis* lozenges. The probiotic treatment led to the total disappearance of all clinical symptoms among all patients. They also had a significant decrease in inflammatory markers nitrite/nitrate, PGE2, matrix metalloproteinase, and saliva IFN-gamma levels.

In another dental school study, *Lactobacillus reuteri* ATCC 55730 or placebo was given to 120 young adults through straw or lozenge daily for 3 weeks. *Streptococcus mutans* were significantly reduced in both probiotic groups as compared to the placebo group and before treatment (Caglar *et al.* 2006).

Researchers at Japan's Tohoku University Graduate School of Dentistry (Shimauchi *et al.* 2008) treated 66 human volunteers with freeze-dried *Lactobacillus salivarius* WB21 lozenge tablets or a placebo for 8 weeks. Periodontal testing confirmed that the probiotic group had significantly greater improvements in plaque index and probing pocket depth compared to the placebo group and before treatment.

Researchers from Turkey's Yeditepe University dental school (Caglar *et al.* 2008) gave 24 healthy young adult volunteers ice-cream containing *Bifidobacterium lactis* Bb-12 or a placebo ice cream for 40 days. Salivary *Streptococcus mutans* counts were significantly reduced in the probiotic ice cream group compared to the placebo group and before treatment.

Scientists from the University of Copenhagen (Twetman *et al.* 2009) gave three groups either chewing gum with placebo or two strains of *Lactobacillus reuteri* for 10 minutes a day for two weeks. Their gums were examined and given immunoassays for gingivitis inflammation. Bleeding on probing was significantly less among the probiotic groups. TNF-alpha and IL-8 significantly decreased among the probiotic group. IL-1beta also decreased during the chewing period. The researchers concluded that, "The reduction of pro-inflammatory cytokines in GCF may be proof of principle for the probiotic approach combating inflammation in the oral cavity."

Researchers from the Institute of Dentistry at the University of Helsinki (Näse *et al.* 2001) investigated the effect of *Lactobacillus rhamnosus* GG on dental caries. Milk without *Lactobacillus rhamnosus* GG was given to 594 children ages 1 to 6 years old. The probiotic group had significantly less dental caries and significantly lower mutans streptococcus counts by the end of the study—especially among the 3- to 4-year-olds.

Scientists from the Universidad Nacional Autónoma de Mexico (Bayona *et al.* 1990) gave 245 seven-year-old children chewable tablets of either pyridoxine (vitamin B6) with heat-killed probiotics (streptococci and lactobacilli) or tablets with pyridoxine once a week for 16 weeks. Four evaluations were made over a two-year period from the beginning of the study. There was a 42% reduction of dental caries among the probiotic group compared to the placebo group.

Scientists from Sweden's Malmö University (Krasse *et al.* 2006) gave *Lactobacillus reuteri* or placebo to 59 patients with moderate to severe gingivitis. After 2 weeks of treatment, the gingival index and plaque index were established from measurements of two teeth surfaces and from saliva. The average gingival index and plaque index was significantly lower in the *L. reuteri* probiotic groups. The researchers concluded that, "*Lactobacillus reuteri* was efficacious in reducing both gingivitis and plaque in patients with moderate to severe gingivitis."

Finnish researchers from the University of Helsinki (Ahola *et al.* 2002) found that the long-term consumption of milk containing *Lactobacillus rhamnosus* GG significantly reduced dental caries. They found this same effect from probiotic cheese ingestion. To illustrate this later effect, the researchers gave 74 young adults a placebo or 60 grams of probiotic cheese per day for three weeks. There were significantly lower salivary *Streptococcus mutans* counts among the probiotic cheese group.

Italian scientists (Petti *et al.* 2001) gave healthy volunteers either yogurt with *Streptococcus thermophilus* and *Lactobacillus bulgaricus* or non-probiotic ice cream for 8 weeks. The probiotic group had lower levels of salivary *Streptococcus mutans* than the control group. However, *L. bulgaricus* was only transiently detected in the oral cavity, indicating that it did not colonize well within the mouth [in contrast with observations of other species such as *L. reuteri*].

Bacterial Infections

We have already discussed how probiotics can conquer and reduce colonies of a multitude of bacteria. Please refer to previous chapters on these mechanisms. Here we will illustrate these with some of the clinical research.

In a German (Mohan *et al.* 2006) study, 69 preterm infants were given placebo or *Bifidobacterium lactis* Bb12. The probiotic supplementation reduced cell counts of enterobacteria and clostridia while increasing counts of bifidobacteria.

Scientists from the Huddinge University Hospital in Sweden (Sullivan *et al.* 2003) compared the antibiotic clindamycin with probiotic yogurt containing *Bifidobacterium lactis* and *Lactobacillus* F19 on twenty-four people. One week of clindamycin treatment was compared to 14 days of probiotic treatment. Bacteria levels of *Bacteroides fragilis, Escherichia coli* and other gram-positive microorganisms were significantly lower in both treatment groups, but healthy probiotic levels were significantly higher among the probiotic group following the treatments.

Researchers from New Zealand's University of Otago (Dierksen *et al.* 2007) gave 219 children *Streptococcus salivarius*-supplemented milk for either 2 days or 9 days. At the beginning of the treatment, a significant number of the children had higher levels of infective *Streptococcus pyrogenes* (which can lead to strep throat and necrotizing fasciitis) populations on the tongue. Following probiotic supplementation, increased levels of salivaricin (produced by *Streptococcus salivarius*) was found among the probiotic group. This antibiotic substance produced by *Streptococcus salivarius* significantly inhibits *Streptococcus pyogenes*.

Scientists from Turkey's Celal Bayar University (Akil *et al.* 2006) gave *Saccharomyces boulardii* to 24 children aged 3-16 years old. *E. coli* colonies per gram in the children's feces declined from 384,625 to 6,283 following probiotic treatment.

The Gastroenterology Unit of the UK's Scarborough General Hospital (Jain *et al.* 2004) studied 90 patients admitted into its intensive care unit for sepsis (internal bacterial infection). Half were given a placebo and half were given a probiotic blend of *Lactobacillus acidophilus* La5, *Bifidobacterium lactis* Bb 12, *Strepto-*

coccus thermophilus and *Lactobacillus bulgaricus* plus prebiotic oligofructose. After one week of treatment, nasogastric aspirate testing showed that the probiotic group had significantly lower incidence of pathogenic bacteria compared to the placebo group (43% versus 75%). The probiotic group also had fewer multiple pathogenic microorganisms (39% versus 75%).

Scientists from the Department of Nutrition at Spain's Universidad Completeness de Madrid (Jimenez *et al.* 2008) studied 20 women with staphylococcal mastitis in a randomized placebo-controlled study. The probiotic group was given *Lactobacillus salivarius* CECT5713 and *Lactobacillus gasseri* CECT5714 (both originally isolated from breast milk) for 4 weeks, and the control group was given a placebo. After 30 days, staphylococcal counts within the probiotic group were significantly lower than the control group (2.96 log(10) CFU/ml versus 4.79 log(10) CFU/ml). Furthermore, *L. salivarius* and *L. gasseri* were also isolated from the breast milk of 6 of the 10 women in the probiotic group. After 14 days of treatment, there were no clinical signs of mastitis observed within the probiotic group. Mastitis persisted among the placebo group.

Eighty burn patients from an Argentina hospital burn unit (Peral *et al.* 2009) had infected second- and third-degree burns, along with non-infected third-degree burns. They were given topical applications of probiotic *Lactobacillus plantarum* or silver sulphadiazine (SD-Ag). (SD-Ag is a typical antimicrobial paste used to prevent infection in burns, along with adverse side effects.) Among both infected and non-infected burns, *L. plantarum* prevented wound infection, and promoted wound granulation healing equal to or better than SD-Ag, without the side effects.

Researchers from the University of Paris (Schiffrin *et al.* 1997) gave 28 volunteers either *Lactobacillus acidophilus* or *Bifidobacterium bifidum* strain Bb12. Phagocytosis (removal) of *Escherichia coli* was enhanced in both probiotic groups.

Ukrainian scientists (Marushko 2000) examined 77 children with streptococcal tonsillitis. They found that the infections were symptomized by a reduction in "tonsil colony resistance." Their trial determined that *L. acidophilus* provided a "highly efficient means of treating tonsillitis of streptococcal etiology."

Irritable Bowel Syndrome and Crohn's

IBS is one of those diseases that physicians like to qualify as an autoimmune disease. As we've discussed earlier, the concept that the body's immune system is attacking itself for no reason is not logical. There are reasons the immune system might target cells from within the body. These can range from the cells being damaged by environmental toxins, endotoxins, oxidative (free) radicals, viruses, to the immune system itself being damaged. How do probiotics intermix within these possibilities?

The research illustrates that probiotics directly attack foreign invaders like bacteria, viruses and fungi, often before they can damage the cells of the intestinal walls. Probiotics can also bind to oxidative radicals formed by many types of toxins. Probiotics will also line the intestinal cells, creating a barrier for toxins to enter the blood. They secrete lactic acid and other biochemicals that prevent endotoxic microorganisms from flourishing. Probiotics will also signal the immune system with the identities of pathogens, and then assist in their eradication.

Deficiencies of probiotics in the intestines usually result in overgrowths of pathogenic microorganisms like *Clostridia* spp., *E. coli*, *H. pylori* and *Candida* spp. These damage the cells of the intestinal wall and produce endotoxins that poison intestinal cells. In addition, a lack of probiotics means that food will not be properly broken down, as probiotics help break down many large food molecules into bioavailable nutrients. This means the intestinal cells will become under-nourished too.

Toxins from our foods will also more easily reach the intestinal wall cells without the protective agency that probiotics provide. For this reason, the intestinal cells have more exposure to various toxic chemicals from our foods and environment, including pesticides, herbicides and preservatives. These can damage intestinal cells to the point where they do not function normally. They can also mutate through adaptation to toxin exposure. Toxin exposure and subsequent genetic alteration can cause the immune system to launch an inflammatory attack on intestinal cells, in an effort to rid them from the body. This can result in the inflammation and pain associated with Crohn's and IBS.

Here is some research supporting these conclusions:

Researchers from the Medical University of Warsaw (Gawrońska *et al.* 2007) investigated 104 children who had functional dyspepsia, irritable bowel syndrome, or functional abdominal pain. They gave the children either placebo or *Lactobacillus rhamnosus* GG. for 4 weeks. The probiotic group had overall treatment success (25% versus 9.6%) compared to the placebo group. The IBS probiotic group had even more treatment success compared to the placebo IBS group (33% versus 5%). The probiotic group also had significantly reduced pain frequency.

French researchers (Drouault-Holowacz *et al.* 2008) gave probiotics or a placebo to 100 patients with irritable bowel syndrome. Between the first and fourth weeks of treatment, the probiotic group had significantly less abdominal pain (42% versus 24%) than the placebo group.

Resesearchers from Poland's Curie Regional Hospital (Niedzielin *et al.* 2001) gave *Lactobacillus plantarum* 299V or placebo to 40 IBS patients. IBS symptoms significantly improved for 95% of the probiotic patients versus just 15% of the placebo group.

Forty IBS patients took *Lactobacillus acidophilus* SDC 2012, 2013 or a placebo for four weeks in research at the Samsung Medical Center and Korea's Sungkyunkwan University School of Medicine (Sinn *et al.* 2008). The probiotic group had a 23% reduction in pain and discomfort while the placebo group showed no improvement.

Scientists from Italy's University of Parma (Fanigliulo *et al.* 2006) gave *Bifidobacterium longum* W11 or rifaximin (an IBS medication) to 70 IBS patients for two months. The probiotic patients reported a fewer symptoms and greater improvement than the rifaxmin patients. The researchers commented: "The abnormalities observed in the colonic flora of IBS suggest, in fact, that a probiotic approach will ultimately be justified."

Researchers from the University of Helsinki (Kajander *et al.* 2008) treated 86 patients with IBS with either a placebo or a combination of *Lactobacillus rhamnosus* GG, *L. rhamnosus* Lc705, *Propionibacterium freudenreichii* subsp. *Shermanii* JS and *Bifidobacterium animalis* subsp. *lactis*. After 5 months, the probiotic group had a significant reduction of IBS symptoms, especially with respect to distension and abdominal pain. The researchers concluded that, "this multispecies probiotic seems to be an effective and safe option to alleviate symptoms of irritable bowel syndrome, and to stabilize the intestinal microbiota."

Scientists from the Canadian Research and Development Centre for Probiotics and The Lawson Health Research Institute in Ontario (Lorea Baroja *et al.* 2007) studied 20 IBS patients, 15 Crohn's patients, 5 ulcerative colitis patients, and 20 healthy volunteers. All subjects were given a yogurt supplemented with *Lactobacillus rhamnosus* GR-1 and *L. reuteri* RC-14 for 30 days. IBS inflammatory markers were tested in the bloodstream. CD4(+) CD25(+) T-cells increased significantly among the probiotic IBS group. Tumor necrosis factor (TNF)-alpha(+)/interleukin (IL)-12(+) monocytes decreased for all the groups except the IBS probiotic group. Myeloid DC decreased among most probiotic groups, but was also stimulated in IBS patients. Serum IL-12, IL-2(+) and CD69(+) T-cells also decreased in probiotic IBS patients. The researchers also concluded that, "Probiotic yogurt intake was associated with significant anti-inflammatory effects..."

Researchers from the General Hospital of Celle (Plein and Hotz 1993) gave *Saccharomyces boulardii* or placebo to 20 Crohn's disease patients with diarrhea flare-ups. After ten weeks, the probiotic group had a significant reduction in bowel movement frequency compared with the control group. The control group's bowel movement frequency rose in the tenth week and then subsided to initial frequency levels—consistent with flare-ups.

In another study from Finland (Kajander *et al.* 2005), a placebo or combination of *Lactobacillus rhamnosus* GG, *L. rhamnosus* LC705, *Bifidobacterium breve* Bb99 and *Propionibacterium freudenreichii* subsp. *shermanii* JS was given to of 103 patients with IBS. The total symptom score (abdominal pain + distension + flatulence + borborygmi) was 7.7 points lower among the probiotic group. This represented a 42% reduction in the symptoms of the probiotic group compared with a 6% reduction of symptoms among the placebo group.

In a study from Yonsei University College of Medicine in Korea (Kim *et al.* 2006), 40 irritable bowel syndrome patients were given either a placebo or a combination of *Bacillus subtilis* and *Streptococcus faecium* for four weeks. The severity and frequency of abdominal pain decreased significantly in the probiotic group.

Researchers from Sweden's Lund University Hospital (Nobaek *et al.* 2000) gave 60 patients with irritable bowel syndrome either a placebo or daily rose-hip drink with *Lactobacillus plantarum* for four weeks. Enterococci levels increased among the placebo group were unchanged in the test group. Flatulence was significantly reduced among the probiotic group compared with the placebo group. At a 12-month follow-up, the probiotic group maintained significantly better overall GI symptoms and function than the placebo group.

New York scientists (Hun 2009) gave 44 IBS patients either a placebo or *Bacillus coagulans* GBI-30 for 8 weeks. The probiotic group experienced significant improvements in abdominal pain and bloating symptoms versus the placebo group.

Scientists at Ireland's University College in Cork (O'Mahony *et al.* 2005) studied 77 irritable bowel syndrome patients with abnormal IL-10/IL-12 ratios—indicating a proinflammatory, Th1 status. The patients were given a placebo, *Lactobacillus salivarius* UCC4331 or *Bifidobacterium infantis* 35624 for eight weeks. IBS symptoms were logged daily and assessed weekly. Tests included quality of life, stool microbiology, and blood samples to test peripheral blood mononuclear cell release of inflammatory cytokines interleukin (IL)-10 and IL-12. Patients who took *B. infantis* 35624 had a significantly greater reduction in abdominal pain and discomfort, bloating and distention, and bowel movement difficulty, compared to the other groups. IL-10/IL-12 ratios—indicative of Th1 proinflammatory metabolism—were also normalized in the probiotic *B. infantis* group.

Researchers from the Umberto Hospital in Venice in Italy (Saggioro 2004) studied probiotics on seventy adults with irritable bowel syndrome. They were given 1) a placebo; 2) a combination of *Lactobacillus plantarum* and *Bifidobacterium breve*; or 3) a combination of *Lactobacillus plantarum* and *Lactobacillus acidophilus* for four weeks. After 28 days of treatment, pain scores measuring different abdominal regions decreased among the probiotic groups by 45% and 49% respectively, versus 29% for the placebo group. The IBS symptom severity scores decreased among the probiotic groups after 28 days by 56% and 55.6% respectively, versus 14% among the placebo group.

Sixty-eight patients with irritable bowel syndrome were treated at the TMC Hospital in Shizuoka, Japan (Tsuchiya *et al.* 2004) with either placebo or a combination of *Lactobacillus acidophilus*, *Lactobacillus helveticus* and *Bifidobacteria* for twelve weeks. The probiotic treatment was either "effective" or "very effective" in more than 80% of the IBS patients. In addition, less than 5% of the probiotic group reported the treatment as "not effective," while more than 40% of the placebo patients reported their placebo treatment as "not effective." The probiotic group also reported significant improvement of bowel habits.

Researchers from Britain's University of Manchester School of Medicine (Whorwell *et al.* 2007) gave a placebo or *Bifidobacterium infantis* 35624 to 362 primary care women with irritable bowel syndrome in a large-scale, multicenter study. After four weeks of treatment, *B. infantis* was significantly more effective than the placebo in reducing bloating, bowel dysfunction, incomplete evacuation, straining, and the passing of gas.

Scientists from Denmark's Hvidovre Hospital and the University Hospital of Copenhagen (Wildt *et al.* 2006) gave 29 colitis-IBS patients either *Lactobacillus acidophilus* LA-5 and *Bifidobacterium animalis* subsp. *lactis* BB-12, or a placebo for twelve weeks. The probiotic treatment group had a decrease in bowel frequency from 32 per week to 23 per week. Furthermore, the probiotic group had an average reduction in the frequency of liquid stools from 6 days per week to 1 day per week.

Scientists at Poland's Jagiellonian University Medical College (Zwolińska-Wcisło *et al.* 2006) tested 293 ulcer patients, 60 patients with ulcerative colitis, 12 patients with irritable bowel syndrome and 72 patients with other gastrointestinal issues. Compared to placebo, *Lactobacillus acidophilus* supplementation resulted in a lessening of symptoms, a reduction of fungal colonization, and increased levels of immune system cytokines TNF-alpha and IL-1 beta.

Medical researchers from Finland's University of Helsinki (Kajander *et al.* 2007) sought to understand the mechanism of probiotics' proven ability to reduce IBS symptoms. They gave either a placebo or a combination of *Lactobacillus rhamnosus* GG, *Lactobacillus rhamnosus* Lc705, *Propionibacterium freudenreichii* subsp. *shermanii* JS and *Bifidobacterium breve* Bb99 to 55 irritable bowel syndrome patients. After six months of treatment, composition of feces and intestinal microorganism content illustrated a significant drop in glucuronidase levels in the probiotic group compared to the placebo group. The researchers concluded that there was a complexity of different factors, and so far unknown mechanisms explaining "the alleviation of irritable bowel syndrome symptoms by the multispecies probiotic."

Digestion Problems

Chronic digestive problems, which include bloating, indigestion, and cramping are often symptoms of IBS, Crohn's disease or colitis. These diseases (IBS, etc.) are also typically accompanied by chronic pain and intestinal inflammation, however. Occasional indigestion, bloating and cramping is often associated with a developing case of dysbiosis caused by antibiotic use, poor diet, or an overgrowth of specific pathogenic microorganisms. Enzyme deficiency can be caused by probiotic deficiencies. Probiotics produce a number of enzymes, including protease and lypase—necessary for the break down of proteins and fats. Poor digestion is often the result of a lack of these and other enzymes. Gastrointestinal difficulties in general are often caused by dysbiosis. This can include an overgrowth of yeasts, pathogenic bacteria or both. Here are a few of the many studies showing that digestion can improve with probiotic use:

French researchers (Guyonnet *et al.* 2009) gave *Bifidobacterium lactis* DN-173010 with yogurt strains to 371 adults reporting digestive discomfort for 2 weeks. 82.5% of the probiotic group reported improved digestive symptoms compared to 2.9% of the control group.

Another group of French scientists (Diop *et al.* 2008) gave 64 volunteers with high levels of stress and incidental gastrointestinal symptoms either a placebo or *Lactobacillus acidophilus* Rosell-52 and *Bifidobacterium longum* for three weeks. At the end of the three weeks, the stress-related gastrointestinal symptoms of abdominal pain, nausea and vomiting decreased by 49% among the probiotic group.

Allergies and Eczema

Allergies have been increasing over the past few decades. Modern medical research is puzzled with this progression. Why are suddenly more people becoming allergic to the plants and pollens that have surrounded humans for thousands of years? This is a huge topic, but we do know from the research that the lack of healthy probiotic colonies is at least a contributing factor.

Probiotics mechanisms have been increasingly connected to inflammatory and allergic responses. They play a critical role in maintaining the epithelial barrier function of the intestinal tract. Allergies appear to increase with intestinal permeability. Without an adequate intestinal barrier, larger food molecules, endotoxins and microorganisms can enter the bloodstream more easily. These increase the body's total toxin burden, making it more sensitive to environmental inputs such as pollen.

Research from Sweden's Linköping University (Böttcher *et al.* 2008) gave *Lactobacillus reuteri* or a placebo to 99 pregnant women from gestational week 36 until infant delivery. The babies were followed for two years after birth, and analyzed for eczema and allergen sensitization and immunity markers. Probiotic supplementation lowered TGF-beta2 levels in mother's milk and babies' feces and slightly increased IL-10 levels in mothers' colostrum. Lower levels of TGF-beta2 are associated with lower sensitization and lower risk of IgE-associated eczema.

German researchers (Grönlund *et al.* 2007) tested 61 infants and mother pairs for allergic status and bifidobacteria levels from 30-35 weeks of gestation and from one-month old. Every mother's breast milk contained some type of bifidobacteria, with *Bifidobacterium longum* found most frequently. However, only the infants of allergic, atopic mothers had colonization with *B. adolescentis*. Allergic mothers also had significantly less bifidobacteria in their breast-milk versus non-allergic mothers. Infants of allergic mothers also had less bifidobacteria in the feces than did infants from non-allergic mothers.

Japanese scientists (Xiao *et al.* 2006) gave 44 patients with Japanese cedar pollen allergies *Bifidobacterium longum* BB536 for 13 weeks. The probiotic group had significantly decreased symptoms of rhinorrhea (runny nose) and nasal blockage versus the placebo group. The probiotic group also had decreased activity among plasma T-helper type 2 (Th2) cells and increased activity among Japanese cedar pollen-specific IgE. The researchers concluded that the results, "suggest the efficacy of BB536 in relieving JCPsis symptoms, probably through the modulation of Th2-skewed immune response."

Researchers from the Wellington School of Medicine and Health Sciences at New Zealand's University of Otago (Wickens *et al.* 2008) studied the association between probiotics and eczema in 474 children. Pregnant women took either a placebo, *Lactobacillus rhamnosus* HN001, or *Bifidobacterium animalis* subsp *lactis* strain HN019 starting from 35 weeks gestation, and their babies received the same treatment from birth to 2 years old. The probiotic infants given *L. rhamnosus* had significantly lower incidence of eczema compared with infants taking the placebo. There was no significant difference between the *B. animalis* group and the placebo group, however.

Researchers from Japan's Kansai Medical University Kouri Hospital (Hattori *et al.* 2003) gave 15 children with atopic dermatitis either *Bifidobacterium breve* M-16V or a placebo. After one month, the probiotic group had a significant improvement of allergic symptoms.

Japanese scientists (Ishida *et al.* 2003) gave a drink with *Lactobacillus acidophilus* strain L-92 or a placebo to 49 patients with perennial allergic rhinitis for eight weeks. The probiotic group showed significant improvement in runny nose and watery eyes symptoms, along with decreased nasal mucosa swelling and redness compared to the placebo group. These results were also duplicated in a follow-up study (2005) of 23 allergy sufferers by some of the same researchers.

Researchers from Tokyo's Juntendo University School of Medicine (Fujii *et al.* 2006) gave 19 preterm infants placebo or *Bifidobacterium breve* supplementation for three weeks after birth. Anti-inflammatory serum TGF-beta1 levels in the probiotic group were elevated on day 14 and remained elevated through day 28. Messenger RNA expression was enhanced for the probiotic group on day 28 compared with the placebo group. The researchers concluded that, "These results demonstrated that the administration of *B. breve* to preterm infants can up-regulate TGF-beta1 signaling and may possibly be beneficial in attenuating inflammatory and allergic reactions in these infants."

Scientists from Britain's Institute of Food Research (Ivory *et al.* 2008) gave *Lactobacillus casei* Shirota (LcS) to 10 patients with seasonal allergic rhinitis. The researchers compared immune status with daily ingestion of a milk drink with or without live *Lactobacillus casei* over a period of 5 months. Blood samples were tested for plasma IgE and grass pollen-specific IgG by an enzyme immunoassay. Patients treated with *Lactobacillus casei* milk showed significantly reduced levels of antigen-induced IL-5, IL-6 and IFN-gamma production compared with the placebo group. Levels of specific IgG also increased and IgE decreased in the probiotic group. The researchers concluded that, "These data show that probiotic supplementation modulates immune responses in allergic rhinitis and may have the potential to alleviate the severity of symptoms."

Researchers from the Skin and Allergy Hospital at the University of Helsinki (Kukkonen *et al.* 2007) studied the role of probiotics and allergies with 1,223 pregnant women carrying children with a high-risk of allergies. A placebo or lactobacilli and bifidobacteria combination with GOS was given to the pregnant women for 2 to 4 weeks before delivery, and their babies continued the treatment after birth. At two years of age, the infants in the probiotic group had 25% less chance of eczema and 34% less chance of contracting atopic eczema.

The same researchers from the Skin and Allergy Hospital and Helsinki University Central Hospital (Kukkonen *et al.* 2009) studied the immune effects of feeding probiotics to pregnant mothers. 925 pregnant mothers were given a placebo or a combination of *Lactobacillus rhamnosus* GG and LC705, *Bifidobacterium breve* Bb99, and *Propionibacterium freudenreichii* ssp. *shermanii* for four weeks prior to delivery. Their infants were given the same formula together with prebiotics, or a placebo for 6 months after birth. During the infants' six-month treatment period, antibiotics were prescribed less often among the probiotic group by 23%. In addition, respiratory infections occurred less frequently among the probiotic group through the two-year follow-up period (even after treatment had stopped) compared to the placebo group (an average of 3.7 infections versus 4.2 infections).

Finnish scientists (Kirjavainen *et al.* 2002) gave 21 infants with early onset atopic eczema a placebo or *Bifidobacterium lactis* Bb-12. Serum IgE concentration correlated directly to *Escherichia coli* and bacteroides counts, indicating the association between these bacteria with atopic sensitization. The probiotic group had a decrease in the numbers of *Escherichia coli* and bacteroides.

Sonicated *Streptococcus thermophilus* cream was applied to the forearms of 11 patients with atopic dermatitis for two weeks. This led to a significant increase of skin ceramide levels, and a significant improvement of their clinical signs and symptoms—including erythema, scaling and pruritus (Di Marzio *et al.* 2003).

Japanese researchers (Odamaki *et al.* 2007) gave yogurt with *Bifidobacterium longum* BB536 or plain yogurt to 40 patients with Japanese cedar pollinosis for 14 weeks. *Bacteroides fragilis* significantly changed with pollen dispersion. The ratio of *B. fragilis* to bifidobacteria also increased significantly during pollen season among the placebo group but not in the *B. longum* group. Peripheral blood mononuclear cells from the patients indicated that *B. fragilis* microorganisms induced significantly more Th2 cell cytokines such as interleukin-6, and fewer Th1 cell cytokines such as IL-12 and interferon. The researchers concluded that, "These results suggest a relationship between fluctuation in intestinal microbiota and pollinosis allergy. Furthermore, intake of BB536 yogurt appears to exert positive influences on the formation of anti-allergic microbiota."

Scientists from the Department of Oral Microbiology at Japan's Asahi University School of Dentistry (Ogawa *et al.* 2006) studied skin allergic symptoms and blood chemistry of healthy human volunteers during the cedar pollen season in Japan. After supplementation with *Lactobacillus casei*, activity of cedar pollen-specific IgE, thymus, chemokines, eosinophils, and interferon-gamma levels all decreased among the probiotic group.

Researchers from the School of Medicine and Health Sciences in Wellington, New Zealand (Sistek *et al.* 2006) determined in a study of *Lactobacillus rhamnosus* and *Bifidobacteria lactis* on 59 children with established atopic dermatitis that food-sensitized children responded significantly better to probiotics than did other atopic dermatitis children.

French scientists (Passeron *et al.* 2006) found that atopic dermatitis children improved significantly after three months of *Lactobacillus rhamnosus* treatment (based on a SCORAD of 39.1 before and 20.7 after).

Scientists from Finland's National Public Health Institute (Piirainen *et al.* 2008) gave a placebo or *Lactobacillus rhamnosus* GG to 38 patients with atopic eczema for 5.5 months—starting 2.5 months before birch pollen season. Saliva and serum samples taken before and after indicated that allergen-specific IgA levels increased significantly among the probiotic group versus the placebo group (using the enzyme-linked immunosorbent assay (ELISA)). Allergen-specific IgE levels correlated positively with stimulated IgA and IgG in saliva, while they correlated negatively in the placebo group. The researchers concluded that the research showed that *L. rhamnosus* GG displayed "immunostimulating effects on oral mucosa seen as increased allergen specific IgA levels in saliva."

Children with cow's milk allergy and IgE-associated dermatitis were given a placebo or *Lactobacillus rhamnosus* GG and a combination of four other probiotic bacteria (Pohjavuori *et al.* 2004). The IFN-gamma by PBMCs at the beginning of supplementation was significantly lower among cow's milk allergy infants. However, those infants receiving *L. rhamnosus* GG significantly increased levels of IFN-gamma among the cow's milk allergy infants.

The British medical publication *Lancet* published a study (Kalliomäki *et al.* 2003) where 107 children with a high risk of atopic eczema were given either a placebo or *Lactobacillus rhamnosus* GG during their first two years of life. Fourteen of 53 children receiving the probiotic developed atopic eczema, while 25 of 54 of the children receiving the placebo contracted atopic eczema by the end of the study.

In a study from the University of Western Australia School of Pediatrics (Taylor *et al.* 2006), 178 children born of mothers with allergies were given either *Lactobacillus acidophilus* or a placebo for the first six months of life. Those given the probiotics showed reduced levels of IL-5 and TGF-beta in response to polyclonal stimulation (typical for allergic responses), and significantly lower IL-10 responses to vaccines as compared with the placebo group. These results illustrated that the probiotics had increased allergen resistance among the probiotic group of children.

Researchers from the Department of Otolaryngology and Sensory Organ Surgery at Osaka University School of Medicine in Japan (Tamura *et al.* 2007) studied allergic response in chronic rhinitis patients. For eight weeks, patients were given either a placebo or *Lactobacillus casei* strain Shirota. Those with moderate-to-severe nasal symptom scores at the beginning of the study given probiotics experienced significantly reduced nasal symptoms compared to the placebo group and before treatment.

Lactose Intolerance

Most nutritionists and physicians assume that lactose intolerance means the person is deficient in the body's production of *lactase*—an enzyme that breaks down milk sugar. New research, however, is indicating that probiotics are as important if not more important for the body's ability to digest milk and break down lactose.

For this very reason, both mother's breast milk and raw cow's milk contain important probiotics that not only furnish lactase: Probiotics also directly digest lactose as part of their own eating regimen. Let's look at the evidence from the research:

Scientists from the University of Buenos Aires (Gaón *et al.* 1995) studied 30 human subjects to see if lactose intolerance could be reduced with probiotics. Milks containing *Lactobacillus casei* and *Lactobacillus acidophilus* or no probiotics were given to the subjects. The subjects drinking the probiotic milk were significantly less likely to have bloating, diarrhea and other symptoms of lactose intolerance than the control group.

Scientists from the Chinese Center for Disease Control and Prevention in Beijing (He *et al.* 2004) gave live probiotic yogurt, heat-treated yogurt or acidified gelled milk (each containing 20 grams of lactose) to 45 lactose-intolerant men. Lactose digestion improved significantly among the live yogurt group compared to the other groups. The researchers concluded that, "The live flora in dairy product could improve lactose digestion in male adult lactose malabsorbers."

Researchers from the University Medical Center Groningen in The Netherlands (He *et al.* 2008) gave *Bifidobacterium longum* and a yogurt enriched with *Bifidobacterium animalis* to 11 lactose-intolerant humans. *Bifidobacterium* levels increased during and after supplementation. *B. animalis* and *B. longum* were not detected before supplementation, but both strains were present in feces during supplementation. They disappeared after supplementation ended. Lactose-intolerance symptoms decreased during supplementation, but resumed following supplementation. The researchers noted that, "supplementation modifies the amount and metabolic activities of the colonic microbiota and alleviates symptoms in lactose-intolerant subjects."

Scientists from the Department of Food Science and Human Nutrition at University of Missouri (Mustapha *et al.* 1997) determined that milk containing *L. acidophilus* was effective in improving lactose digestion and tolerance.

Beta-galactosidase from the yeast *Kluyveromyces lactis* eaten at mealtime with milk and cereal (cornflakes) and an unrefined cereal (bran) reduced lactose intolerance in a Guatamalan study (Solomons *et al.* 1985) of lactose intolerant patients. Exogenous betagalactosidases produced by the probiotic yeast eliminate lactose malabsorption in those deficient in lactase.

Scientists from Alabama's A&M University (Onwulata *et al.* 1989) gave plain yogurt, sweet acidophilus milk, hydrolyzed-lactose milk, or a lactase tablet and whole milk to ten lactose-intolerant humans. They found that the lactase produced by the probiotics in yogurt was "superior to exogenous commercial lactase in alleviating lactose maldigestion."

Scientists from University of Minnesota's Department of Food Science and Nutrition (Jiang *et al.* 1996) gave 15 lactose intolerant patients milk with lactose control milk, or *Bifidobacterium longum* cultured in either lactose or both lactose and glucose. Consumption of milk with lactose-grown *B. longum* resulted in significantly less hydrogen production and flatulence among the patients than the other milks. The researchers concluded that, "milks containing *B. longum* might reduce breath hydrogen response and symptoms from lactose malabsorption when the culture is grown in a medium containing only lactose to induce a higher beta-galactosidase level and increase rate of lactose uptake."

Intestinal Permeability

For years, traditional practitioners described a digestive disorder termed "leaky gut syndrome." This was largely dismissed by the medical establishment as anecdotal and non-existent. In recent years, however, research on intestinal drug absorption by the pharmaceutical industry has confirmed that the lining of the small intestine is subject to alteration, dramatically affecting absorption and permeability. As this research has progressed, it has become apparent that nutrient absorption can be significantly reduced due to permeability alteration. Worse, increased intestinal permeability syndrome (IIPS) may well be implicated in many allergic and arthritic conditions.

These diseases are related to the fact that permeability allows macromolecules—larger peptides, toxins and even invading microorganisms—into the bloodstream. Once these foreigners arrive in the bloodstream, the immune system may activate a variety of inflammatory responses as a defense measure. For example, the invasion of pathogenic microorganisms through the intestinal wall can result in bacterial translocation throughout the body—stimulating inflammatory responses (Baik 2004; Yasuda *et al.* 2006). Illustrating this mechanism, *Blastocystis hominis*, a bacterial pathogen typically found in the intestines, has been found within synovial membranes of arthritic patients (Kruger *et al.* 1994)

The intestinal brush barrier is a complex mucosal layer of enzymes, probiotics and ionic fluid. It forms a protective surface medium over the intestinal epithelium. It also provides an active nutrient transport mechanism. This mucosal layer is stabilized by the grooves of the intestinal microvilli. It contains glycoproteins and other ionic transporters, which attach to nutrient molecules, carrying them across intestinal membranes. Meanwhile the transport medium requires a delicately pH-balanced mix of ionic chemistry able to facilitate this transport of amino acids, minerals, vitamins, glucose and fatty acids. The mucosal layer is policed by billions of probiotic colonies, which help process incoming food molecules, excrete various nutrients, and control pathogens. In the proper mucosal environment, probiotics will produce several B vitamins and potent antibiotics (DeWill and Kudsk 1999).

The brush barrier is a triple-filter that screens for molecule size, ionic nature and nutrition quality. Much of this is performed via four mechanisms existing between the intestinal microvilli: tight junctions, adherens junctions, desmosomes, and of course probiotics. The tight functions form a bilayer interface between cells, controlling permeability. Desmosomes are points of interface between the tight junctions, and adherens junctions keep the cell membranes adhesive enough to stabilize the junctions. These junction mechanisms together regulate permeability at the intestinal wall.

This mucosal brush barrier creates the boundary between intestinal contents and our bloodstream. Should the mucosal layer chemistry become altered, its protective and ionic transport mechanisms become weakened, allowing toxic or larger molecules to be presented to the microvilli junctions. This contact can irritate the microvilli, causing a subsequent inflammatory response. This is now considered a contributing cause of IBS.

This situation also weakens the microvilli junctions, allowing the larger molecules immediate access to the bloodstream.

Intestinal permeability is caused by a number of factors. Alcohol is one of the most irritating substances to the mucosal lining and junctions. In addition, many pharmaceutical drugs, notably NSAIDs, have been identified as damaging to the mucosal chemistry and intestinal junction strength. Foods with high arachadonic fatty acid capability (such as trans-fats and animal meats); low-fiber, high-glucose foods; and high nitrite-forming foods have been suspected for their ability to compromise the intestinal lining. Toxic substances such as plasticizers, pesticides, herbicides, chlorinated water and food dyes are also suspected.

Substances that increase PGE-2 response also negatively affect permeability (Martin-Venegas *et al.* 2006).

In addition, the overuse of antibiotics can cause a die-off of the all-important resident probiotic colonies. When intestinal probiotic colonies are decreased, pathogenic bacteria and yeasts can outgrow probiotic colonies. Pathogenic bacteria growth invades the brush barrier, introducing an influx of endotoxins (the waste matter of these microorganisms) into the bloodstream together with some of the microorganisms themselves.

Holistic doctors have attributed the influx of macromolecules into the bloodstream as a major cause for the increasing occurrence of food allergies in western society. Typically, intestinal barriers let only smaller molecules access to the liver and bloodstream—usually beneficial nutrients. Should larger, undigested food molecules enter the bloodstream—even if from a food consumed for decades—the body's immune system will not recognize them. This can lead to IgA and/or IgE responses, stimulating heightened histamine levels. This in turn can cause skin and/or sinus inflammatory responses.

This scenario is happening more frequently in western society. A food that has been a source of nutrition for many years begins to be identified by the immune system as toxic. This unfortunate circumstance results not only in the possibility of allergic response to some foods: Nutritional deficiencies can also result. Research is finally confirming these mechanisms (Laitinen and Isolauri 2005; Fasano and Shea-Donohue 2005).

Inflammatory responses resulting from IIPS are thus associated with sinusitis, allergies, psoriasis, asthma, arthritis and other inflammatory disorders. Overgrowth of *Candida albicans*, a typical fungal inhabitant of the digestive system at controlled populations, has also been attributed to IIPS. Systemic Candida infections have a route of translocation via IIPS.

The research has supported the link between IIPS and liver damage (Bode and Bode 2003). Alcohol consumption has also been associated with IIPS (Ferrier *et al.* 2006). Alcohol also damages probiotic populations (Bongaerts and Severijnen 2005).

In a study by scientists from China's Qilu Hospital and Shandong University (Zeng *et al.* 2008), 30 irritable bowel syndrome patients with intestinal wall permeability were given either a placebo or a fermented milk beverage with *Streptococcus thermophilus, Lactobacillus bulgaricus, Lactobacillus acidophilus* and *Bifidobacterium longum*. After four weeks, intestinal permeability reduced significantly among the probiotic group.

Researchers from Greece's Alexandra Regional General Hospital (Stratiki *et al.* 2007) gave 41 preterm infants of 27-36 weeks gestation a formula supplemented with *Bifidobacterium lactis* or a placebo. After 7 days, bifidobacteria counts were significantly higher, head growth was greater, and the lactulose/mannitol ratio (a marker for intestinal permeability) was significantly lower after 30 days in the probiotic group as compared to the placebo group. The researchers concluded that, "bifidobacteria supplemented infant formula decreases intestinal permeability of preterm infants and leads to increased head growth."

Granada medical researchers (Lara-Villoslada *et al.* 2007) gave *Lactobacillus coryniformis* CECT5711 and *Lactobacillus gasseri* CECT5714 or a placebo to 30 healthy children after having received conventional yogurt containing *Lactobacillus bulgaricus* and *Streptococcus thermophilus* for three weeks. The supplemented yogurt significantly inhibited *Salmonella cholerasuis* adhesion to intestinal mucins compared to before probiotic supplementation. The probiotic supplementation also increased IgA concentration in feces and saliva.

German scientists (Rosenfeldt *et al.* 2004) gave *Lactobacillus rhamnosus* 19070-2 and *L. reuteri* DSM 12246 or a placebo to 41 children. After six weeks of treatment, the frequency of GI symptoms were significantly lower (10% versus 39%) among the probiotic group as compared to the placebo group. In addition, the lactulose-to-mannitol ratio was lower in the probiotic group, indicating to the researchers that, "probiotic supplementation may stabilize the intestinal barrier function and decrease gastrointestinal symptoms in children with atopic dermatitis."

Researchers from the People's Hospital and the Jiao Tong University in Shangha (Qin *et al.* 2008) gave *Lactobacillus plantarum* or placebo to 76 patients with acute pancreatitis. Intestinal permeability was determined using the lactulose/rhamnose ratio; and organ failure, septic complications and death was also monitored. After 7 days of treatment, microbial infections averaged 38.9% in the probiotic group and 73.7% in the placebo group. 30.6% of the probiotic group colonized potentially pathogenic organisms, as compared to 50% of patients in the control group. The probiotic group also had significantly better clinical outcomes compared with the control group. The researchers concluded that *Lactobacillus plantarum* "can attenuate disease severity, improve the intestinal permeability and clinical outcomes."

Polyps, Diverticulosis and Diverticulitis

Polyps, diverticulosis and diverticulitis are abnormalties within the intestines or colon. They have been associated with Crohn's, IBS and ulcerative colitis, as well as intestinal cancer. They also have been seen forming seemingly without other disease pathologies. Diverticulosis is the bulging of sections of the intestines. When a bulging area weakens and bursts, that is called diverticulitis. A polyp, on the other hand, is a growth on the inside of the intestinal wall. These may be either benign, or cancerous. All of these conditions are associated with intestinal probiotics, because healthy probiotic colonies are essential to the health of the intestinal wall. We can see the evidence from the research:

Scientists from Sweden and Ireland (Rafter *et al.* 2007) gave placebo or *Lactobacillus rhamnosus* GG and *Bifidobacterium lactis* Bb12 to 43 polyp patients (who also had surgery for their removal) for 12 weeks. The probiotics significantly reduced colorectal proliferation and improved epithelial barrier function (reducing intestinal permeability) among the polyp patients. Testing also showed decreased exposure to intestinal genotoxins among the probiotic polyp patient group.

Researchers from The Netherlands' University Hospital Maastricht (Goossens *et al.* 2006) gave *Lactobacillus plantarum* 299v or a placebo to 29 polyp patients twice a day for two weeks. Fecal sample examinations and biopsies were collected during colonoscopy. *L. plantarum* 299v significantly increased probiotic bacteria levels from fecal tests and from rectal biopsies. Ascending colon populations were not significantly greater, however.

Researchers from the Digestive Endoscopy Unit at Italy's Lorenzo Bonomo Hospital (Tursi *et al.* 2008) treated 75 patients with symptomatic diverticulosis. Mesalazine and/or *Lactobacillus casei* DG were given for 10 days each month. Of the 71 patients that completed the study, 66 (88%) were symptom-free after 24 months. The researchers concluded that mesalazine and/or *Lactobacillus casei* were effective in maintaining diverticulosis remission for an extended period, assuming continued treatment.

Ulcers

Just a couple of decades ago, medical scientists and physicians were certain that ulcers were caused by too much acid in the stomach and the eating of spicy foods. This assumption has been debunked over the past two decades as researchers have confirmed that at least 80% of all ulcers are associated with *Helicobacter pylori* infections.

While acidic foods and gastrin produced by the stomach wall are also implicated with symptoms of heartburn and acid reflux, we know that a healthy stomach has a functional barrier that should prevent these normal food and gastric substances from harming the cells of the stomach wall. This barrier is called the mucosal membrane. This stomach's mucosal membrane contains a number of mucopolysaccharides and phospholipids that, together with secretions from intestinal and oral probiotics, protect the stomach cells from acids, toxins and bacteria invasions.

As doctors and researchers work to eradicate *H. pylori,* which infects billions of people worldwide, they are finding that *H. pylori* is becoming increasingly resistant to many of the antibiotics used in prescriptive treatment. Research from Poland's Center of Gastrology (Ziemniak 2006) investigated antibiotic use on *Helicobacter pylori* infections: 641 *H. pylori* patients were given various antibiotics typically applied to *H. pylori.* The results indicated that *H. pylori* had developed a 22% resistance to clarithromycin and 47% resistance to metronidazole. Worse, a 66% secondary resistance to clarithromycin and metronidazole was found, indicating *H. pylori's* increasing resistance to antibiotics.

H. pylori bacteria do not always cause ulcers. In fact, only a small percentage of *H. pylori* infections actually become ulcerative. Meanwhile, there is some evidence that *H. pylori*—like *E. coli* and *Candida albicans*—may be a normal resident in a healthy intestinal tract, assuming it is properly balanced and managed by strong legions of probiotics.

Here are some research data that confirms the ability probiotics have in controlling and managing *H. pylori* overgrowths. Here we will also see probiotics' ability to arrest ulcerative colitis and even mouth ulcers:

Researchers from the Academic Hospital at Vrije University in The Netherlands (Cats *et al.* 2003) gave either a placebo or *Lactobacillus casei* Shirota to 14 *H. pylori*-infected patients for three weeks. Six additional *H. pylori*-infected subjects were used as controls. The researchers determined that *L. casei* significantly inhibits *H. pylori* growth. This effect was more pronounced for *L. casei* grown in milk solution than in the DeMan-Rogosa-Sharpe medium (a probiotic broth developed by researchers in 1960).

Mexican hospital researchers (Sahagún-Flores *et al.* 2007) gave 64 *Helicobacter pylori*-infected patients antibiotic treatment with or without *Lactobacillus casei* Shirota. *Lactobacillus casei* Shirota plus antibiotic treatment was 94% effective and antibiotic treatment alone was 76% effective.

Researchers from the Department of Internal Medicine and Gastroenterology at Italy's University of Bologna (Gionchetti *et al.* 2000) gave 40 ulcerative colitis patients either a placebo or a combination of four strains of lactobacilli, three strains of bifidobacteria, and one strain of *Streptococcus salivarius* subsp. *thermophilus* for nine months. The patients were tested monthly. Three patients (15%) in the probiotic group suffered relapses within the nine months, versus 20 (100%) in the placebo group.

Italian scientists from the University of Bologna (Venturi *et al.* 1999) also gave 20 patients with ulcerative colitis a combination of three bifidobacteria strains, four lactobacilli strains and *Streptococcus salivarius* subsp. *thermophilus* for 12 months. Fecal samples were obtained at the beginning, after 10 days, 20 days, 40 days, 60 days, 75 days, 90 days, 12 months and 15 days after the (12 months) end of the treatment period. Fifteen of the 20 treated patients achieved and maintained remission from ulcerative colitis during the study period.

British researchers from the University of Dundee and Ninewells Hospital Medical School (Furrie *et al.* 2005) gave 18 patients with active ulcerative colitis either *B. longum* or a placebo for one month. Clinical examination and rectal biopsies indicated that sigmoidoscopy scores were reduced in the probiotic group. In addition, mRNA levels for human beta defensins 2, 3, and 4 (higher in active ulcerative colitis) were significantly reduced among the probiotic group. Inflammatory cytokines tumor necrosis factor alpha and interleukin-1alpha were also significantly lower in the probiotic group. Biopsies showed reduced inflammation and the regeneration of epithelial tissue within the intestines among the probiotic group.

Scientists from Italy's Raffaele University Hospital (Guslandi *et al.* 2003) gave *Saccharomyces boulardii* or placebo to 25 patients with ulcerative colitis unsuitable for steroid therapy, for 4 weeks. Of the 24 patients completing the study, 17 attained clinical remission—confirmed endoscopically.

Researchers from Switzerland's University Hospital in Lausanne (Felley *et al.* 2001) gave fifty-three patients with ulcerative *H. pylori* infection milk with *L. johnsonii* or placebo for three weeks. Those given the probiotic drink had a significant *H. pylori* density decrease, reduced inflammation and less gastritis activity from *H. pylori*.

Lactobacillus reuteri ATCC 55730 or a placebo was given to 40 *H. pylori*-infected patients for 4 weeks by researchers from Italy's Università degli Studi di Bari (Francavilla *et al.* 2008). *L. reuteri* effectively suppressed *H. pylori* infection, decreased gastrointestinal pain, and reduced other dyspeptic symptoms.

Scientists from the Department of Internal Medicine at the Catholic University of Rome (Canducci *et al.* 2000) tested 120 patients with ulcerative *H. pylori* infections. Sixty patients received a combination of antibiotics rabeprazole, clarithromycin and amoxicillin. The other sixty patients received the same therapy together with a freeze-dried, inactivated culture of *Lactobacillus acidophilus*. The probiotic group had an 88% eradication of *H. pylori* while the antibiotic-only group had a 72% eradication of *H. pylori*.

Scientists from the University of Chile (Gotteland *et al.* 2005) gave 182 children with *H. pylori* infections placebo, antibiotics or probiotics. *H. pylori* were completely eradicated in 12% of those who took *Saccharomyces boulardii*, and in 6.5% of those given *L. acidophilus*. The placebo group had no *H. pylori* eradication.

Researchers from Japan's Kyorin University School of Medicine (Imase *et al.* 2007) gave *Lactobacillus reuteri* strain SD2112 in tablets or a placebo to 33 *H. pylori*-infected patients. After 4 and 8 weeks, *L. reuteri* significantly decreased and suppressed *H. pylori* in the probiotic group.

In a study of 347 patients with active *H. pylori* infections (ulcerous), half the group was given antibiotics and the other half was given antibiotics with yogurt (*Lactobacillus acidophilus* HY2177, *Lactobacillus casei* HY2743, *Bifidobacterium longum* HY8001, and *Streptococcus thermophilus* B-1). The yogurt plus antibiotics group had significantly more eradication of the *H. pylori* bacteria, and significantly less side effects than the antibiotics group (Kim, *et al.* 2008).

Lactobacillus brevis (CD2) or placebo was given to 22 *H. pylori*-positive dyspeptic patients for three weeks before a colonoscopy by Italian medical researchers (Linsalata *et al.* 2004). A reduction in the UBT delta values and subsequent bacterial load ensued. *L. brevis* CD2 stimulated a decrease in gastric ornithine decarboxylase activity and polyamine. The researchers concluded: "Our data support the hypothesis that *L. brevis* CD2 treatment decreases *H. pylori* colonization, thus reducing polyamine biosynthesis."

Thirty *H. pylori*-infected patients were given either probiotics *Lactobacillus acidophilus* and *Bifidobacterium bifidum* or placebo for one and two weeks following antibiotic treatment by British researchers (Madden *et al.* 2005). Those taking the probiotics had a recovery of normal intestinal microflora, damaged during antibiotic treatment. The researchers also observed that those taking the probiotics throughout the two weeks showed more normal and stable microflora than did those groups taking the probiotics for only one out of the two weeks.

Researchers at the Nippon Medical School in Tokyo (Fujimori *et al.* 2009) gave 120 outpatients with ulcerative colitis either a placebo; *Bifidobacterium longum;* psyllium (a prebiotic); or a combination of *B. longum* and psyllium (synbiotics) for four weeks. C-reactive protein (pro-inflammatory) decreased significantly only with the synbiotic group, from 0.59 to 0.14 mg/dL. In addition, the synbiotic therapy experienced significantly better scores on symptom and quality-of-life assessment.

Scientists from the Department of Medicine at Lausanne, Switzerland's University Hospital (Michetti *et al.* 1999) tested 20 human adults with ulcerative *H. pylori* infection with *L. acidophilus johnsonii*. The probiotic was taken with the antibiotic omeprazole in half the group and alone (with placebo) in the other group. The patients were tested at the start, after two weeks of treatment, and four weeks after treatment. Both groups showed significantly reduced *H. pylori* levels during and just following treatment. However, the probiotic-only group tested better than the antibiotic group during the fourth week after the treatment completion.

Medical scientists from the Kaohsiung Municipal United Hospital in Taiwan (Wang *et al.* 2004) studied 59 volunteer patients infected with *H. pylori*. They were given either probiotics (*Lactobacillus* and *Bifidobacterium* strains) or placebo after meals for six weeks. After the six-week treatment period, the probiotic group "effectively suppressed *H. pylori*," according to the researchers.

In the Polish study mentioned earlier (Ziemniak 2006), 641 *H. pylori* patients were given either antibiotics alone or probiotics with antibiotics. The two antibiotic-only treatment groups had 71% and 86% eradication of *H. pylori*, while the antibiotic-probiotic treatment group had 94% eradication.

Researchers from the Cerrahpasa Medical Faculty at Istanbul University (Tasli *et al.* 2006) gave 25 patients with Behçet's syndrome (chronic mouth ulcers) six *Lactobacillus brevis* CD2 lozenges per day at intervals of 2-3 hours. After one and two weeks, the number of ulcers significantly decreased.

Constipation

Most of us have experienced constipation from time to time. The slow movement of the bowels has been associated with a lack of fiber in the diet and meat-rich diets. Meat of course, is extremely low in fiber, and also moves slowly through the intestines because of its high saturated fat and complex protein makeup. The intestines do not assimilate complex proteins— they need them broken down into amino acids or smaller poly- peptides in order for the body to use them as nutrients. This re- quires significant protease enzymes and other digestive resources. For these reasons and others, animal meats tend to double or triple the time of passage through the digestive tract. This slow passage of meat diets typically causes putrefaction.

Putrefaction means that the food stimulates the growth of pathogenic bacteria colonies. These bacteria become stronger partially because meat is not a typical probiotic food. Probiotics do not like meat, as we'll discuss further later on. Probiotics feed and thrive from vegetable fibers and complex carbohydrates. High fiber meals thus move through the digestive tract more easily for a number of reasons: Fibers provide food for probiot- ics. They bind to cholesterols and speed up intestinal fat metabo- lism (lowering blood cholesterol levels). Fibers also do not attract pathogenic bacteria populations.

As we'll see from the research, probiotics speed up the pas- sage of food through the digestive tract because they assist in the digestive process, and they help reduce pathogenic bacteria populations involved in the putrefaction process.

Italian scientists (Amenta *et al.* 2006) gave *Bifidobacterium longum* W11 + FOS or placebo to 297 chronic constipation pa- tients undergoing a weight loss diet. Constipation was signifi- cantly reduced among patients in the probiotic group.

Researchers from the Taiwan's Keelung Hospital (Bu *et al.* 2007) studied 45 children with chronic constipation. They gave the children a placebo, *Lactobacillus casei* rhamnosus Lcr35, or the laxative magnesium oxide. Those receiving either MgO or the probiotic had higher defecation frequency and treatment success than the placebo group. While there was no statistically signifi- cant difference in effectiveness between the MgO and the probiotic treatment groups, less abdominal pain occurred in the probiotic treatment group than the MgO group.

Scientists from Italy's University of Bologna (Colecchia *et al.* 2006) gave 636 patients diagnosed with IBS with constipation either a placebo, or *Bifidobacterium longum* and a prebiotic for at least 36 days. Patients reporting no bloating increased from 3% to 27%, and reports of no abdominal pain went from 8% to 44% in the probiotic group. Severe symptom frequency dropped significantly, from 63% to 9.5% for bloating, and from 39% to 4% for abdominal pain among the probiotic group. Average stool frequency increased from 2.9 to 4.1 times per week among the probiotic group.

Researchers from the Helsinki University Hospital (Pitkala *et al.* 2008) gave live *Bifidobacterium longum,* live *B. lactis* or inactivated placebo to 209 constipated elderly nursing home residents. The live probiotic groups had significantly increased bowel movement frequency compared to the placebo group. The normal bowel movement level for the *B. longum* group was slightly higher than the *B. lactis* group, but each of the probiotic groups were higher than the placebo group.

We add that significant research (such as Sturtzel *et al.* 2009) has established that plant fibers like oat bran can also significantly decrease constiptation. Fiber plus probiotics: Even better.

Pancreatitis

A variety of studies has shown that the pancreas can be damaged by either pathogenic bacteria endotoxins that leak in from the intestines or pathogenic bacteria themselves (called pancreatic sepsis). Because the pancreas is critical to the production of insulin and other key biochemicals that assist in energy metabolism, an infected pancreas can mean the shut down or slow down of energy production, strength and vitality.

Medical researchers from Hungary's Petz Aladár Teaching Hospital (Oláh *et al.* 2003; Kecskés *et al.* 2003) gave *Lactobacillus plantarum* 299 or placebo to 45 patients with acute pancreatitis who had arrived at the hospital within 48 hours after the onset of symptoms. Twenty-two of the pacreatitis patients received treatment with live *L. plantarum,* and 23 received heat-killed *L. plantarum* 299. Infected pancreatic necrosis and abscesses were found in only 1 of the 22 patients in the live probiotic group, versus 7 of the 23 among the inactivated probiotic group. The mean hospital stay was 13.7 days in the live probiotic group versus 21.4 days among the inactivated probiotic group. The researchers concluded that, "Supplementing *Lactobacillus plantarum* 299 is an effective tool to prevent pancreatic sepsis, to reduce the number of operations and length of stay. The only patient who developed sepsis in the treatment group did so eight days after the treatment had been discontinued."

In terms of the mechanisms of pancreatitis mechanisms, the researchers also confirmed that, "Colonization of the lower gastrointestinal tract and oropharynx, mostly with gram-negative but sometimes also gram-positive bacteria is known to precede the contamination of the pancreatic tissue by a few days."

Kidney Stones and Kidney Disease

Kidney stones and kidney disease is rampant within the western world because of a combination of poor diet, high levels of chemical toxins in our foods and water, and dysbiosis. Our kidneys must push out many toxins and this puts a strain on the glomeruli within the kidneys. Especially tough on the kidneys is increased levels of uric acid, which is often caused by high dietary protein content. Yes, the western world eats too much protein. While our bodies only require 30-50 grams of a mixture of essential amino acids per day, the western diet often contains 75-150 grams of protein per day. This overabundance of protein in the form of amino acids and polypeptides produces excess uric acid, which can build up in cells throughout the body. Gout, for example, is the build up of uric acid crystals within the joints.

Excess uric acid can overload the kidneys. Combined with fatty acids and minerals, several different types of kidney stones can form as a result of uric acid overload. This combined with an overload of chemical toxins from our foods and water, and endotoxins from an overgrowth of pathogenic bacteria, can be dangerous to the kidneys.

Probiotics can be helpful for excess uric acid and kidney problems because they help reduce levels of endotoxins produced by pathogenic bacteria. These endotoxins increase the acidity of the blood, and thus increase the rate of uric acid crystals (oxalate) formation. Endotoxins also produce an additional toxic load the kidneys must filter and deal with.

Researchers from the S. Orsola University Hospital's Department of Nephrology in Bologna, Italy (Campieri *et al.* 2001) gave a combination of *L. acidophilus*, *L. plantarum*, *L. brevis*, *S. thermophilus*, and *B. infantis* to six patients with idiopathic calcium-oxalate urolithiasis and mild hyperoxaluria (oxalate kidney stones) for four weeks. They were tested for urine oxalate levels before and during treatment. Probiotic treatment resulted in a significant reduction in urine oxalate (from SD levels of 55.5 to 28.3 in thirty days) and a significant reduction in fecal oxalate excretion.

Researchers from the Mayo Clinic (Lieske *et al.* 2005) gave 10 patients with chronic fat malabsorption, calcium oxalate kidney stones, and hyperoxaluria *Lactobacillus* probiotics or placebo for three months. Patients treated with probiotics had a 20% drop in urinary oxalate excretion after the three months. The study authors also noted that other research concluded that people with inflammatory bowel disease have a 10 to 100 times increased risk of nephrolithiasis (kidney disease) related to hyperoxaluria (high uric acid). The researchers concluded that, "Manipulation of gastrointestinal (GI) flora can influence urinary oxalate excretion to reduce urinary supersaturation levels. These changes could have a salutary effect on stone formation rates."

Researchers from the Jefferson Medical College (Simenhoff *et al.* 1996) gave 8 kidney hemodialysis patients *Lactobacillus acidophilus* in an attempt to curtail the progression of small bowel bacteria overgrowth—a typical occurrence in end-stage kidney failure. Probiotic treatment lowered serum dimethylamine (a marker for kidney disease) levels from 224 to 154 micrograms/dl and nitrosodimethylamine (another kidney disease marker) from 178 to 83 ng/kg. Serum albumin, body weight, appetite and muscle mass also improved.

Researchers (Schulman 2006) at Vanderbilt University School of Medicine found in a preliminary clinical study that *Bifidobacterium longum* slowed progression of chronic kidney disease.

Vaginosis and Vaginitis

The vagina is lined with probiotic bacteria just as the mouth is. These bacteria protect the woman's internal tissues and organs from being overwhelmed by pathogenic bacteria, yeasts and other pathogens. Without a balance of probiotic bacteria, overgrowths can take place easily. Normal colonies within a healthy vagina include lactobacilli, *Gardenella vaginalis*, *Candida albicans* and other microorganisms—all existing in balance.

Vaginosis is the alteration of the normal microbiological ecology. Vaginitis is an overgrowth of pathogenic bacteria, and their resulting infection. Two common infective microorganisms within the vagina are *Candida albicans* and *Trichomonas vaginalis*. The use of antibiotics, antiseptics and chemical toxins can stress probiotic populations, allowing overgrowths to take place.

Vaginitis can easily lead to urinary tract infections as pathogenic bacteria colonies expand. Vagina microbial infection is often symptomized by stinging sensations and a fishy odor from the vagina. As we'll discuss later and as indicated in the research, internal supplementation (through the mouth) and external application (into the vagina) both have been shown to help replenish the probiotic populations within the vagina.

Estrogen production can also be a factor. Researchers from Israel's HaEmek Medical Center (Colodner *et al.* 2003) determined from research that, "The lack of lactobacilli in the vagina of postmenopausal women due to estrogen deficiency plays an important role in the development of bacteriuria."

Researchers from the School of Medicine at Italy's Università degli Studi di Siena (Delia *et al.* 2006) treated 60 healthy women with vaginosis with either a vaginal suppository containing *Lactobacillus acidophilus* or a suppository containing *Lactobacillus acidophilus* and *Lactobacillus paracasei* F19. At the end of three months of treatment—and again three months afterward—both groups showed significant improvement in vaginosis, a significant reduction in vaginal pH, and significant decrease in vagina odor.

In a study from the University of Milan (Drago *et al.* 2007), forty women with vaginosis took a douche with *Lactobacillus acidophilus* for six days. After treatment, only 7.5% of the women still had the vaginosis. The odor typical in vaginosis discontinued in all the women, and the pH went to normal levels of 4.5 in 34 of the 40 women.

Scientists from the University of Western Ontario (Reid *et al.* 2001) gave 42 women oral encapsulated *Lactobacillus rhamnosus* GR-1 plus *Lactobacillus fermentum* RC-14 probiotics, or *L. rhamnosus* GG orally for 28 days. Vaginal flora—normal in only 40% of the cases—resolved to healthy flora in 90% of the women in the GR-1 group, and the 7 of 11 women with microbial vaginosis at the beginning of the study were resolved within a month. *L. rhamnosus* GG did not have an effect.

In a similar study (Reid *et al.* 2003), 64 women were given placebo or *Lactobacillus rhamnosus* GR-1 and *Lactobacillus fermentum* RC-14 daily for 60 days. The treatment resulted in the restoration from microbial vaginosis microflora to normal lactobacilli-colonized microflora in 37% of the women treated with the probiotic, versus only 13% among the placebo group.

Researchers from Israel's Central Emek Hospital (Shalev *et al.* 1996) gave 46 microbial vaginosis patients either yogurt with live *L acidophilus* or a placebo for several months. The probiotic group had significantly less vaginosis than the control group.

Researchers from Sweden's Uppsala University Hospital (Hallén *et al.* 1992) gave 60 women infected with microbial vaginosis either a placebo or *Lactobacillus acidophilus*. At the end of the study, 16 of the 28 women treated with lactobacilli had normal vaginal wet smear results while no improvement occurred among the 29 women treated with the placebo. Infective vagina bacteroides were eliminated from 12 of 16 women in the probiotic group.

Italian scientists (Cianci *et al.* 2008) investigated the use of *Lactobacillus rhamnosus* GR-1 and *Lactobacillus reuteri* for the treatment and prevention of vaginosis and microbial vaginitis. Fifty women with diagnosed microbial vaginosis and vaginitis took either a placebo or an oral combination of *Lactobacillus rhamnosus* GR-1 and *Lactobacillus reuteri* RC-14 following antibiotic therapy. The researchers found that 92% of the patients significantly benefited from the probiotic treatment.

Scientists from Brazil's Universidade de Sao Paulo (Martinez *et al.* 2009) gave 64 women with microbial vaginosis tinidazole with placebo or with a combination of oral *Lactobacillus rhamnosus* GR-1 and *Lactobacillus reuteri* RC-14 daily for four weeks. The probiotic group experienced a cure rate of 87%, while the placebo group experienced a 50% cure rate. Normal vagina flora resumed in 75% of the probiotic group and in only 34% of the placebo group. This research team (2009) found similar results in another study on 55 women with vulvovaginal candidiasis.

Researchers from the Department of Obstetrics and Fetomaternal Medicine at Austria's Medical University of Vienna (Petricevic and Witt 2008) tested 190 women with microbial vaginosis. They were given either placebo or topical plus oral *Lactobacillus rhamnosus* after antibiotic treatment for 7 days.

Sixty-nine of 83 (or 83%) in the probiotic group significantly improved, versus 31 of the 88 women (35%) in the placebo group.

Another study done by researchers from the Medical University of Vienna (Petricevic *et al.* 2008) gave *Lactobacillus rhamnosus* GR-1 and *Lactobacillus reuteri* RC-14 or placebo to 72 postmenopausal women with vaginosis for seven days. Both the placebo group and the probiotic group had received antibiotic treatment for seven days prior. Four weeks after treatment concluded, 60% (21 of 35) of the probiotic group demonstrated a significant improvement, while only 6 of the 37 non-probiotic subjects (16%) showed the same level of improvement.

Candida Infections

Candida albicans is a normal inhabitant of the intestinal tract and several other locations throughout the body. Complications arise when *Candida* populations have been allowed to grow beyond their normal levels. Lower probiotic populations allow these fungi to easily grow beyond their healthy levels, infecting the intestines, vagina and many other parts of the body. The consumption of probiotics can help return *Candida* back to its normal population levels, as probiotics manage and control their colonies by secreting chemicals that limit their growth.

Researchers from Long Island Jewish Medical Center's Division of Infectious Diseases (Hilton, *et al.* 1992) studied thirty-three patients with vulvovaginal candida infections. Infection rates decreased by a third among patients consuming an eight-ounce yogurt (orally) with *Lactobacillus acidophilus* for six months. The infection rate was 2.54 per six months in the control group versus 0.38 in the yogurt group, while *Candida* spp. colonization rates were 3.23 in the control group versus only 0.84 in the yogurt group—through the six-month testing period.

Premature Births

As mentioned in the section on vaginosis, the vagina contains a complex combination of various probiotics and eubiotic organisms. In a balanced state, these not only can defend against invaders: They can help manage the pH environment and the balance of hormones and nutrients. As the research will show, the baby thrives from a particular environment within the womb of the mother. Healthy colonies of probiotics help create and maintain that environment. Dysbiosis, on the other hand, produces a toxic environment for both the mother and the baby.

In a German study (Hoyme and Saling 2004), among 381 pregnant women, seventy-three were identified as risk cases for premature birth. Fifty-eight of the high-risk cases were treated with a *Lactobacillus* preparation (applied to the vagina) and 24 were treated with clindamycin (antibiotic) cream. (Others refused any therapy). The prematurity rate was 8% in the probiotic group, versus 12% in the control group. Furthermore, the probiotic group resulted in 0.3% versus 3.3% of their neonates being classified as "very early" premature infants.

Seventy-three preterm infants were given either *Lactobacillus* probiotics or placebo at the Ewha Womans University Hospital (Lee *et al.* 2007) between March 2003 and July 2004. The Infants with gestational ages less than 37 weeks were given *Lactobacillus acidophilus* orally, mixed with breast milk or put into formula. After two weeks, the infants given the probiotics had significantly improved feeding tolerance.

Low Birth Weights

When a baby is born premature, they are also likely to have a very low birth weight. Very low birth weights are considered one of the leading causes of death among premature infants. The problem is that with a low birth weight, the infant struggles to maintain metabolic and enzymatic activity. The key to stimulating weight among a low birth weight infant is thus proper digestion and assimilation of nutrients. The problem often with a premature infant is that they have yet to develop the mechanisms for the production of digestive aids such as bile, enzymes and gastrin that properly break down foods. This is where pro-biotics come into play. Probiotics help the body break down nu-trients, and help stimulate the production of enzymes. Probiotics also help stimulate healthy mucosal membranes and intestinal barriers. Let's review some research that supports this:

Japanese scientists from the Osaka Medical Center (Kitajima *et al.* 1997) gave *Bifidobacterium breve* or placebo to 91 very low birthweight infants for eight weeks and followed up for three years. At two weeks of age, colonization rates of the adminis-tered bacteria were 73% versus 12% among the control group. The probiotic group showed significantly fewer abnormal ab-dominal signs and better weight gain than the control group.

Scientists from China's Medical University (Lin *et al.* 2005) gave 367 infants with very low birth weights either *Lactobacillus acidophilus* and *Bifidobacterium infantis* with their breast milk or breast milk alone. Those given the probiotics were five times less likely to contract necrotizing enterocolitis—a frequent disorder among very low birth weights—than did the control group. Fur-thermore, the probiotic group had no severe cases of necrotizing enterocolitis while the control group suffered six severe cases.

Another study—this time a multicenter study of 435 in-fants—from some of the same researchers (Lin *et al.* 2008) showed that death and necrotizing enterocolitis among low birth weight newborns significantly decreased for newborns who were supplemented with probiotics.

Researchers from Israel's Shaare Zedek Medical Center and the Faculty of Medicine from Hebrew University (Bin-Nun *et al.* 2005) gave a combination of *Bifidobacteria infantis*, *Streptococcus thermophilus* and *Bifidobacteria Bifidus* or a placebo to 145 low birth-weight infants. Necrotizing enterocolitis was significantly lower in the probiotic group than in the placebo group (4% ver-sus 16%). Fewer severe cases also occurred in the probiotic in-fants. Three of the 15 babies who developed necrotizing enterocolitis died—with all the deaths sadly occurring among the placebo infants.

Researchers from the Neonatal Intensive Care Unit at Italy's Azienda Ospedaliera Regina Anna Hospital (Manzoni *et al.* 2006) studied 180 neonates with very low birth weight. They gave either a placebo or oral *Lactobacillus rhamnosus* beginning on the first three days of life through the earlier of six weeks or until discharge. The infants' health was tracked over a 12-month period. Incidence of *Candida* infections among the infants was significantly lower in the probiotic group (23.1% vs. 48.8%).

Researchers from India's Kolkata Medical College (Samanta *et al.* 2009) showed that death and necrotizing enterocolitis among low birth weight newborns significantly decreased for those newborns given probiotics.

Scientists from the University of Tartu's Department of Pediatrics in Estonia (Vendt *et al.* 2006) investigated *Lactobacillus rhamnosus* GG supplementation among normal healthy infants. One hundred and twenty healthy infants under two months old were given a probiotic-supplemented formula or a non-probiotic formula until the age of six months. Weight, length and head circumference were measured monthly. Combined, these measurements were all greater among the probiotic infants. In other words, those infants given *Lactobacillus rhamnosus* GG with their feeding formula grew significantly faster than those not given probiotics!

Baby Colic

Colic is the incessant crying of a baby, often resulting in radical oxygen reduction and further complications. Modern medicine does not understand colic very well. There are a number of theories as to its cause. Many believe that microbial infections are the main cause. Others feel that it has more to do with nutrition or perhaps their environment. Studies with probiotics give us another perspective on this mystery.

Researchers at Johns Hopkins University School of Medicine (Saavedra *et al.* 2004) gave a *Bifidobacterium lactis* and *Streptococcus thermophilus* combination or a placebo to 118 infants (average age 2.9 months) for 210 days. The probiotic group had a significantly lower frequency of colic and irritability, and a lower need (frequency) for antibiotics than did the placebo group.

Italian researchers from the University of Bari Policlinico (Indrio *et al.* 2008) gave 30 preterm newborns either a placebo or *Lactobacillus reuteri* ATCC 55730 for 30 days. Newborns fed with probiotics had a significant reduction in regurgitation and mean daily crying time. Probiotic newborns also had more stools compared with the placebo group. Gastric emptying rates significantly increased, and fasting antral area (inverse marker for digestive health) was significantly reduced among the newborns given *L. reuteri* and the breast-fed newborns, versus the placebo groups.

Researchers from Italy's Regina Margherita Children's Hospital (Savino *et al.* 2007) gave either simethicone (colic medication) or *Lactobacillus reuteri* to 90 children with infantile colic. After 28 days, 39 patients (95%) responded positively among the probiotic group, while only three patients (7%) responded positively among the simethicone group. Most breastfed infants improved colicky symptoms in the *L. reuteri* group within 1 week of treatment.

Ear Infections

Most of us would laugh at the prospect that probiotics would help or prevent ear infections. Think again.

Scientists from Sweden's University of Gothenburg (Skovbjerg *et al.* 2009) studied the effect of probiotic treatment on secretory otitis media—an ear infection with fluid in the middle ear cavity. Sixty children suffering from chronic secretory otitis media who were scheduled for tympanostomy tube insertion were given a nasal spray of placebo, *Streptococcus sanguinis* or *Lactoba-*

cillus rhamnosus for 10 days prior to surgery. "Complete or significant clinical recovery" occurred in 7 of 19 patients treated with *S. sanguinis*; in 3 of 18 patients treated with *L. rhamnosus*; and in 1 of 17 of the placebo patients.

Anorexia Nervosa

Modern medicine classifies anorexia nervosa as a psychological disorder. Most people who have anorexia nervosa, however, will likely say otherwise. While many who have anorexia nervosa are characterized by an excessive compulsion to lose weight or appear attractive to others, there are also biological components to the disease. A person with anorexia has also lost the physical desire to eat. A person with anorexia nervosa also has the same lack of physical desire, but this will be accompanied by anxiety about their weight or appearance. In both cases, other things are more important than eating. This, however, has a biological component because a proper appetite has not been developed in either case. In a healthy person, there may also be anxiety about appearance, but there will still be hunger.

Anxiety stresses more than just our minds. When we are anxious, our adrenal glands begin to produce stress chemicals such as adrenaline. This is accompanied by a mechanism that shuts down our appetite. Our vagus nerve is stimulated in a way that decreases our stomach's output of mucopolysaccharides and gastrin. Our salivary glands slow down their production of enzymes. Our body's appetite for food is physically put aside, in order to make way for the needs of the moment. This is mirrored by a stimulated immune system, which further shuts down the body's ability to produce the right chemistry for digestion and appetite.

This stress, and the resulting chemistry, also deters the growth of our probiotics. In fact, as we will find, stress directly reduces probiotic populations. And with this reduction comes a reduced ability to digest foods. It is a vicious cycle, in which our innocent probiotic helpers become victims of our mind's anxieties, and our body's physical response to stress.

Illustrating this connection, scientists from Spain (Nova *et al.* 2006) gave yogurt with *L. bulgaricus* and *S. thermophilus* or placebo to 16 anorexia nervosa (AN) adolescent patients and 15 healthy adolescents for 10 weeks. Blood lymphocyte subsets were examined through quantitative testing. These revealed that the probiotics stimulated increased CD8+ subset and IFN-gamma production in both HA and AN probiotic groups. The researchers concluded: "The findings suggest that the inclusion of yogurt in the refeeding therapy of AN patients may exert positive effects on the immunological markers related to the nutritional status of these patients, such as the CD4+/CD8+ ratio and the production of IFN-gamma by lymphocytes."

Keratoconjunctivitis

Keratoconjunctivitis is an inflammation of the conjunctiva of the eyes. As in most forms of inflammation, this can be due to toxins, microbial infection, stress or lacrimal dryness (malfunction of lacrimal gland). Pathogenic endotoxins and bacteria are often the cause of these issues. The immune system launches an inflammatory attack to resolve the situation and clear out the toxins or pathogens. This is where probiotics can come in. There is some evidence that probiotics might also be dwelling within the lacrimal fluids of eye. This is supported by research showing the improvement of keratoconjunctivitis with probiotics:

Medical researchers from the University of Rome (Iovieno *et al.* 2008) gave seven patients with vernal keratoconjunctivitis eye drops with *Lactobacillus acidophilus* for four weeks. After treatment, 6 of 7 showed significant improvement of clinical symptoms after two weeks of treatment. These symptoms included itching, photophobia and burning. In addition, clinical signs—such as conjunctiva hyperemia, chemosis, secretion, Trantas dots and superficial punctuate keratitis—all showed significant improvement among the patients after the four weeks of probiotic treatment.

Immunosuppression

Immunosuppression may be a long word, but it really is very simple: The immune system has been overburdened and compromised. This is the result of a myriad of combined effects. The chart below itemizes a few of the causes of immunosuppression:

Source	Toxin
Antacids	Heavy Metals
Antiperspirant	Aluminum
Bottled Water	Plasticizers (see also tap water)
Carpets, rugs	Molds, dander, lice, PC-4, latex
Cigarette Smoke	Carbon monoxide, nicotine, aldehydes, ketones
Cosmetics	Aluminum, phosphates and chemicals
Dental Fillings	Mercury, alloys, various chemicals
Dish soap	Perfumes, dyes, phosphates
Electric Blankets	EMFs, PC-4, various toxins
Food	MSG, preservatives, trans-fats, pesticides, arachadonic acids
Soaps and Shampoos	Perfumes, chemicals, phosphates
House	Radon, Formaldehyde, Pollen, Dust, Mold, Dander
Householder cleaners	chlorine, various phosphates
Indoor Light	Fluorescent Lights
Industrial Plant or Freeway	Lead, mercury, carbon monoxide
IUDs	Copper
Laundry soaps	Perfumes, dyes, phosphates
Old pillows	Lice eggs, dander, molds
Paints	Lead, arsenic, cadmium, various toxins

Pesticides	Neurotoxins, poisons
Pets	240 infectious diseases & parasites (65 from dogs/39 from cats)
Pipes	Lead, copper, deposits
Pools and spas	Chlorine, various carbonates
Appliances and X-rays	Electromagnetic frequencies
Restaurants	Parasites, pesticides, trans-fats
Pans	Aluminum, copper, lead
Shampoo	Perfumes, chemicals, phosphates
Stoves, Fireplaces	Carbon monoxide, arsenic, soot
Tap Water	Giardia, *Cryptosporidium*, pesticides, nitrates, pharmaceuticals
Toothpaste	Fluoride, p. glycol and sweeteners
Work environment	Various toxins
Microorganisms	See tables in Chapter One

For each of these toxins, the liver and immune system must launch a variety of macrophages, T-cells and B-cells to break them apart and escort them out of the body. This means that each toxin represents an additional load the immune system must carry.

We might compare this to moving dirt. A small handful of dirt can be carried around easily, and dispersed without much effort. However, a truckful of dirt is another matter completely. What do we do with a truckful of dirt? If we dumped it on our lawn, we'd have a hill of dirt blowing around and blocking us from getting in and out of the house.

This is a useful comparison because while our bodies can handle a small amount of toxins quite easily, modern society is increasingly dumping toxic 'dirt' into our atmosphere, water and foods, effectively inundating our bodies by the 'truckload.'

The modern world's toxin soup burdens an immune system trying to adapt and clean up each toxin and its damaging effects.

Many of today's diseases, including arthritis, cancer, heart disease, Alzheimer's Disease and many others, are connected to immunosuppression due to the overload of toxins. Even a person's response to viruses or even the common cold may be related to the level of immunosuppression. An immunosuppressed person will likely get much sicker and can even die from an infection that a healthy body would throw off in a few days.

What does this have to do with probiotics? Lots. Probiotics are miniature workers that help carry our immune loads. They block many toxins and pathogens from getting into our bodies in the first place. Then they break down many toxins if they do get in. They will bind to and escort toxins out of the body by latching onto them like little bulldogs. More importantly, probiotics will stimulate the immune system. Let's look at the evidence:

Researchers from the Osaka University Graduate School of Medicine (Morimoto *et al.* 2005) studied 99 addicted smokers for three weeks. They were given either a fermented milk containing *Lactobacillus casei* or a placebo. NK cell activity among peripheral blood mononuclear cells was measured before and after taking probiotics, and before and after smoking. NK cell activity reduced with the number of cigarettes smoked. However, NK cell activity was significantly higher after taking probiotics.

Ten healthy volunteers and nine volunteers with ileostomy underwent gastroscopy or ileoscopy along with *Lactobacillus reuteri* ATCC 55730 supplementation for 28 days (Valeur *et al.* 2004). After probiotic supplementation, gastric mucosal histiocyte numbers had reduced, and duodenal B-lymphocyte numbers had increased. *L. reuteri* supplementation also induced a significantly higher level of CD4-positive T-lymphocytes within the ileal epithelium. The scientists concluded that *L. reuteri* "is associated with significant alterations of the immune response in the gastrointestinal mucosa."

Researchers from Canada's Memorial University of Newfoundland (Arunachalam *et al.* 2000) gave *Bifidobacterium lactis*

HN019 to 25 healthy elderly volunteers for 6 weeks. Interferon-alpha levels and polymorphonuclear cell phagocytic capacity increased substantially. The probiotic group also experienced enhanced phagocyte-mediated bactericidal activity. The researchers said that, "The results demonstrate that dietary consumption of *B. lactis* HN019 can enhance natural immunity in healthy elderly subjects, and that a relatively short-term dietary regime is sufficient to impart measurable improvements in immunity that may offer significant health benefits to consumers."

Researchers from the Teikyo University School of Medicine in Japan (Araki *et al.* 1999) gave *Bifidobacterium breve* YIT4064 or placebo to 19 infants for 28 days. After the treatment period, the probiotic group experienced significantly modulated levels of immunoglobulin IgA.

Scientists from The Netherlands (van Baarlen *et al.* 2009) gave living or heat-killed *Lactobacillus plantarum* to healthy adults. Biopsies were taken from the mucosa of their intestinal duodenums before and after the treatment period. These examinations indicated significantly different NF-kappaB-dependent pathways after the consumption of living *L. plantarum* bacteria in different growth phases. These mucosal gene expression patterns and cellular-immunity pathways correlated with increased immune tolerance among the subjects.

Pediatric medical researchers from the University of Bari (Indrio *et al.* 2007) gave a placebo or a combination of *Bifidobacterium breve* C50 and *Streptococcus thermophilus* 065 to 60 newborns. In addition, a control group of thirty newborns who were exclusively breastfed was included. Fecal pH of the breast-fed group and the probiotic formula group were similar — and significantly lower than the placebo group during the first few days of treatment. Meanwhile, thymus size was significantly larger in the probiotic group compared to the standard formula-placebo group. The probiotic group thymus sizes were similar to those of the breast-fed newborns.

Researchers from the Department of Immunology at Juntendo University's School of Medicine in Tokyo (Takeda and Okumura 2007) determined in a three-week study on 19 elderly volunteers that *Lactobacillus casei* strain Shirota significantly increased natural killer cell activity. This effect was particularly significant among those patients who began the study with low NK-activity levels.

Researchers at Belgium's University Hospital Leuven (De Preter *et al.* 2004) determined in a in a study of 19 healthy volunteers that *Lactobacillus casei* suppressed the production of toxic metabolites within the body.

Russian scientists (Bliakher *et al.* 2005) gave sickly children a *Lactobacillus* supplement, and assessed immune responses. They found the probiotics stimulated the immune system by modulating the activities of interferon, phagocytes, and cytokines among the children.

Researchers from the Department of Clinical Sciences at Spain's University of Las Palmas de Gran Canaria (Ortiz-Andrellucchi *et al.* 2008) studied the ability of *Lactobacillus casei* DN114001 to modulate immunity factors among lactating mothers and their babies. *L. casei* or a placebo was given to expecting mothers for six weeks. T helper-1 and T helper-2 (Th1/ Th2) levels were tested from breast-fed colostrum, early milk (10 days) and mature milk (45 days). Allergic episodes among the newborns were also observed throughout their first six months of life. Among the probiotic group, T and B lymphocyte levels were increased, and natural killer cells were significantly increased. Levels of the pro-inflammatory cytokine TNF-alpha was decreased in maternal milk. Significantly fewer gastrointestinal upsets occurred among the breast-fed children of the probiotic mother group as well.

Immune system suppression has been observed in students stressed during examinations. Spanish scientists (Marcos *et al.* 2004) gave 136 university students either a placebo or milk fermented with *Lactobacillus casei* for three weeks before examinations and during the three-week examination period. The probiotic group showed a significant increase in lymphocytes during the six weeks—which decreased among the placebo group. CD56+ cells decreased in the placebo group but stayed consistent in the probiotic group. The researchers concluded that *Lactobacillus casei* was "able to modulate the number of lymphocytes and CD56+ cells in subjects under academic examination stress."

Researchers from New Zealand's Massey University (Gill *et al.* 2001) investigated using probiotics to enhance risk of infectious and noninfectious disease and age-related lymphocyte activity. Twenty-seven elderly volunteers consumed low-fat and low-lactose milk supplemented with *Lactobacillus rhamnosus* HN001 or *Bifidobacterium lactis* HN019 for 3 weeks. The proportion of CD56+ lymphocytes among peripheral circulation was higher after probiotic supplementation. CD4+ and CD25+ activity increased among the probiotic group. PBMC tumor killing activity also increased. Subjects more than 70 years of age and those who were immune-suppressed experienced significantly greater improvements in immune system parameters than did the other subjects.

Researchers from the College of Medicine at National Taiwan University (Chiang *et al.* 2000) gave *Bifidobacterium lactis* HN019 to 50 persons aged from 41 to 81 years old. The probiotic group had significantly enhanced PMN cell phagocytosis and NK-cell tumor killing activity. The increases leveled off after *B. lactis* supplementation was discontinued, but still remained above the values at the beginning of the study.

Researchers from the Russia State Medical University in Moscow (Korschunov *et al.* 1996) studied five men who received accidental, uneven and high-dose, whole-body gamma-irradiation from exposure to an unshielded radiation source. Feces examinations 9-12 days after irradiation showed low numbers of anaerobes and high counts of enterobacteria and staphylococci in four of the five patients. All five were treated with ampicillin and gentamicin with oral nystatin starting 4-7 days after irradiation. Three were also given an antibiotic-resistant strain of *Bifidobacterium longum* for 30 days starting 10-12 days following irradiation while the other two received a placebo. After three weeks after irradiation, *B. longum* was observed in their feces, and this continued in the following weeks. In comparison, the two placebo patients' fecal flora was dominated by enterobacteria, including *Klebsiella, Staphylococcus* and *Serratia* spp. These showed resistance to multiple antibiotics. These pathogens were not found in the *B. longum*-treated group. One of the patients in the placebo group died. The other one continued to show high fecal counts of enterobacteria and staphylococci. The researchers concluded that, "Probiotic treatment with this antibiotic-resistant strain of *B. longum* may be of benefit in the treatment of radiation sickness, aiding normalization of the fecal flora and inhibiting colonization and overgrowth with opportunist pathogens."

Scientists from Bulgaria's National Oncological Centre (Krusteva *et al.* 1997) gave *Lactobacillus bulgaricus* to 78 patients who underwent combined chemotherapy and had subsequent moderate leukopenia (lack of white blood cells—a classic sign of immunosuppression). A recovery of WBC count (values above 3000) took place in all probiotic patients within three to five days. No infectious or febrile complications resulted from subsequent chemotherapy and probiotic treatment.

German scientists (Rayes *et al.* 2002) tested 172 patients who just had major abdominal surgery or liver transplantation with either conventional nutrition, *Lactobacillus plantarum* 299, or heat inactivated lactobacilli. Following treatment, bacteria infection after liver, gastric or pancreas resection was 31% in the conventional nutrition group, 13% in the heat-inactivated probiotic group and 4% in the probiotic group. Among the 95 liver transplant patients, 48% of the conventional nutrition group patients developed infections; while 34% of the inactive probiotic group and 13% of the live probiotic group developed infections (cholangitis and pneumonia were the most frequent). The use and duration of antibiotic therapy among the patients was also significantly shorter in the live probiotics group.

Cancer

At first glance, it might seem outlandish to propose that probiotics can prevent or even cure cancer. However, a number of studies—*in vitro, in vivo* and clinical research on humans—have confirmed that probiotics inhibit tumor cells through possibly several mechanisms. These include the inhibition of the enzymes beta-glucosidase, beta-glucuronidase, and urease. These enzymes have been conclusively associated with increased tumor cell growth in hundreds of other studies. Beta-glucuronidase, for example, seems to convert certain molecules into procarcinogens. In addition to blocking these enzymes, probiotics also stimulate natural killer cells and cytotoxic T-cells that eliminate tumor cells. Let's examine some of the clinical research:

Researchers from the Gastrointestinal Research Department of the University Hospital Gasthuisberg in Belgium (De Preter *et al.* 2008) determined, in study of 53 healthy volunteers, that probiotic combinations such as *Lactobacillus casei* Shirota, *Bifidobacterium breve* and *Saccharomyces boulardii* were able to significantly reduce beta-glucuronidase activity in the colon. Beta-glucuronidase activity, as mentioned above, has been associated with reducing carcinogenic metabolites within the colon.

Thirty-eight healthy volunteers were given either a placebo or a combination of *Lactobacillus rhamnosus* and *Propionibacterium freudenreichii* subsp. *shermanii* JS for four weeks (Hatakka *et al.* 2008). The probiotic group had significantly lower levels of beta-glucosidase activity and urease activity compared to the placebo group.

Researchers from the Department of Urology and the Faculty of Medicine from the University of Tokyo (Aso *et al.* 1995) conducted a study of 138 patients with superficial transitional cell carcinoma of the bladder following transurethral resection surgery. They gave patients either *Lactobacillus casei* or a placebo. The probiotic groups showed significantly better results than the placebo group in all cases except for those with recurrent multiple tumors—where there was no significant difference between the probiotic and placebo group. The researchers concluded that *L. casei* "was thus safe and effective for preventing recurrence of superficial bladder cancer."

In an earlier study by some of the same medical researchers from the University of Tokyo (Aso and Akazan 1992), *Lactobacillus casei* or placebo was given to 48 patients with bladder cancer following transurethral resection. The recurrence-free interval was significantly prolonged by the probiotic treatment, to 350 days, compared to the 195 days in the control (non-probiotic) group.

Scientists from Japan's Osaka University Medical School (Masuno *et al.* 1991) tested *L. casei* on 76 patients with malignant pleural effusions secondary to lung cancer. Response rates for treatment with intrapleural doxorubicin plus the probiotic was 73.7%, while the response rate without the probiotic was 39.5% in the control group treated with doxorubicin alone. The probiotic group also had a significantly longer survival rates than the control group. The probiotic group also had significantly greater improvement in symptoms such as chest pain, chest discomfort, and anorexia than the control group.

Researchers from the Graduate School of Medical Sciences at Japan's Kyushu University (Naito *et al.* 2008) studied 207 patients diagnosed with superficial bladder cancer who underwent transurethral resection, followed by treatment with the pharmaceutical epirubicin. One hundred of the patients were randomized to receive *Lactobacillus casei* every day for one year in addition to the epirubicin treatment. The lack of recurrence in three years was significantly higher among the probiotic group (74.6% versus 59.9%).

Japanese researchers (Matsumoto and Benno 2004) gave yogurt with *Bifidobacterium lactis* LKM512 or placebo to seven healthy adults for two weeks. The yogurt group showed increased anticarcinogenic fecal spermidine levels and significantly reduced mutagenicity (the likelihood of mutations) levels (48% versus 79%) compared to the placebo group.

Scientists from the Taipei Medical College Hospital and the College of Medicine at Taiwan's National University of Taiwan (Sheih *et al.* 2001) gave *Lactobacillus rhamnosus* HN001 in low-fat milk or lactose-hydrolyzed low-fat milk for 3 weeks to elderly adults with an average age of 64. PMN phagocytic activity increased among the two probiotic groups by 19% and 15%, respectively. NK cell tumor-killing activity increased by 71% and 147%. These declined after the supplement periods, but remained higher than before treatment.

Researchers from the School of Health Sciences and Nursing at the University of Tokyo (Ohashi *et al.* 2002) studied 180 cases of bladder cancer and 445 control subjects in a multi-center (7) study. Subjects given fermented milk products with *Lactobacillus casei* had a significantly reduced risk of bladder cancer, depending upon the frequency and dosage.

This Japanese study (Okamura *et al.* 1989) tested *L. casei* with and without mitomycin on patients with stomach cancer. The probiotic was given either alone or with the mitomycin C with 29 patients enrolled. The positive response rate was 60% for the probiotic group and 70% for those given both the probiotic and mitomycin. The researchers concluded that this probiotic strain "might be a useful therapeutic agent against carcinomatous peritonitis of gastric cancer whether used alone or in combination with mitomycin."

Japanese researchers (Okawa *et al.* 1993) investigated a combined therapy of radiation with heat-killed *Lactobacillus casei* on

228 patients with Stage IIIB cervical cancer. They found that probiotic combination therapy significantly increased tumor regression, and prolonged survival rates. It also increased the relapse-free intervals of patients. In addition, they found that radiation-induced leukopenia was significantly less among the probiotic group.

Researchers from the Japan's Hyogo College of Medicine (Ishikawa *et al.* 2005) studied the association between fiber, probiotics and colorectal tumors. They gave 398 volunteers who were currently free from tumors but who had at least two colorectal tumors removed in the past either wheat bran, *L. casei*, a combination of both or neither. The *L. casei* groups showed a significantly lower risk of atypia—cell abnormality—compared with the non-probiotic groups.

Researchers from the University of Wuerzburg's medical college (Bartram *et al.* 1994) concluded from several clinical studies that, "diet-induced changes in the colonic microflora seem to play a role in colon carcinogenesis."

Scientists from Sweden's Karolinska Institute (Rafter *et al.* 2007) examined probiotics' ability to inhibit colon cancer in a twelve-week study mentioned earlier. Thirty-seven colon cancer patients were given either a placebo or a combination of *Lactobacillus rhamnosus* GG and *Bifidobacterium lactis* Bb12 with FOS. The probiotic group had significant changes in fecal flora. Fecal *Bifidobacterium* and *Lactobacillus* levels increased, while *Clostridium perfringens* levels decreased. The probiotic group also had significantly reduced colorectal proliferation; and fecal water from this group could better induce necrosis (killing) of tumor cells. The probiotic group also had increased interleukin-2 production from peripheral blood mononuclear cells, and increased interferon gamma production among the cancer patients—all anticarcinogenic mechanisms.

German scientists (Roller *et al.* 2007) tested a combination of probiotics and prebiotics in colon cancer patients. Thirty-four colon cancer patients who underwent colon resection were given either a placebo or capsules with *Lactobacillus rhamnosus* GG and *Bifidobacterium lactis* Bb12 with inulin/FOS. At six weeks and twelve weeks, researchers found that IL-2 cytokines from activated PBMCs increased significantly, IFN-gamma production capacity increased—both anticarcinogenic mechanisms.

Researchers from Japan's Nagoya University Graduate School of Medicine's Department of Surgery (Sugawara *et al.* 2006) studied 101 patients with liver/biliary cancer following liver surgery. NK-cell activity and lymphocyte counts were significantly higher following surgery, and pro-inflammatory cytokine IL-6 decreased significantly in the probiotic group. C-reactive protein (another pro-inflammatory marker) also significantly decreased among the probiotic group. Postoperative infectious complications occurred in 30.0% of the placebo group and 12.1% of the probiotic group.

Medical researchers from the Institute of Immunology and Faculty of Medicine of Bratislava's Comenius University (Ferencík *et al.* 1999) summarized the benefits of lactic acid bacteria: "These include: 1. Lactose digestion, improvement of diarrheal disorders (including traveler's diarrhea), prophylaxis of intestinal and urogenital infections—as a result of formation or reconstruction of a balanced indigenous microflora. 2. Inhibition of the mutagenicity of the intestinal contents and reduction of the incidence of intestinal tumors. 3. Immunomodulatory effects resulting in the improved host resistance. 4. Depression of the serum cholesterol level." These effects were seen during the researchers' nine-week clinical study. Lyophilized *Enterococcus faecium* M-74 in the form of waffles were used. Among the probiotic subjects, beta-D-glucuronidase in stool samples was reduced compared to those of the placebo group. The probiotic group also showed higher production of reactive oxygen species-neutralizing superoxide and peripheral neutrophils. This also accompanied an increase in IgG from peripheral blood mononuclear cells, increased activity from myeloperoxidase and elastase in peripheral neutrophils. The researchers concluded that, "intake of *E. faecium* M-74 in the form of waffles may have a significant immunostimulatory effect on both phagocytosis performed by neutrophils and antibody production."

HIV/AIDS

Aren't we taking the benefits of probiotics a bit too far now? Actually, no. HIV stands for *Human Immunodeficiency Virus.* AIDS stands for *Acquired Immune Deficiency Syndrome.* What are these, then? Once again, we find the immune system has become compromised—this time after being overburdened by viral infection on top of the other toxic burdens our modern society throws at our bodies.

To clarify, we must ask why there is a great disparity between survival rates of HIV-infected persons. One HIV sufferer may live for decades, while another may be diagnosed with AIDS and die within a year. The difference lies in the efficiency and strength of the immune system. The big questions include: How capable is the immune system at suppressing the virus? How well does the immune system interact with its various components to keep its defenses up?

In a study from Italy's University of Milan, researchers (Clerici *et al.* 2996) examined 26 long-term HIV-positive patients who were not progressing into AIDS, and compared them to 28 HIV-positive patients who were progressing rapidly and 24 HIV-seronegative controls (who tend to live longer). They found that cytokine levels, cytokine production rates and the surface marker expression of peripheral blood mononuclear cells (PBMCs) related directly to whether the patient had a longer survival rate. Let's review the research more analytically:

HIV Patient Type	Cytokine levels
Nonprogressing (long term survival, not progressing into AIDS)	Reduced IL-2 Reduced IFN-gamma Increased IL-4 Increased IL-10 Decrease in CD57, CD4, CD7 lymphocytes
Rapidly progressing	Increased IL-2 Increased IFN-gamma Decreased IL-4 Decreased IL-10 Increase in CD57, CD4, CD7 lymphocytes
Seronegative (long term survival)	same as Nonprogressing

We can see here that the ability to fight off the virus is directly related to the immune system's effectiveness and efficiency. Cytokines—the immune system's targeted signaling devices—are produced by the immune system. When it is healthy and not overburdened, it has greater capacity to produce effective cytokines. Lymphocytes with CD programming are specifically programmed to attack certain types of invaders. The production of certain CD lymphocytes indicate an overwhelmed and weaked immune response.

What does this have to do with probiotics? Everything. Probiotics stimulate the production of cytokines, often specific to the type of infection a person might have. This may seem surprising. How would a tiny probiotic know what is attacking the body, and how can it relay that information to the immune system?

Probiotics are conscious living organisms. They want to survive. Like any living being, when their survival is threatened, they get serious. They begin to devise strategies to increase their colonies' chance of survival.

Probiotics are also smart organisms. They utilize several means of communication, including biochemical ligands, biophoton signaling, and a colony communication process called quorum sensing. The orchestrated illumination of tiny algae that appears on the ocean at night is an example of quorum sensing. Even yeasts have these facilities (Chwirot and Popp 1991).

As we have seen from the research covered previously, probiotics often stimulate the production of cytokines specific to the particular ailment. Because the same species of probiotics are stimulating different immune responses for different ailments, this can only mean that the probiotics are responding in an intelligent manner to specific threats to their host.

This ability of probiotics to stimulate specific immune responses in specific disease pathologies has been illustrated in the probiotic research with HIV/AIDS sufferers:

Brazilian scientists (Trois *et al.* 2008) gave a placebo or a formula containing *Bifidobacterium bifidum* and *Streptococcus thermophilus* to 77 HIV-infected children. The average CD4 count in the probiotics group increased by +118 cells mm(-3), while CD4 decreased in the placebo group by -42 CD4 cells mm(-3). Stool consistency also increased among the probiotics group. The researchers concluded: "Our study showed that probiotics have immunostimulatory properties and might be helpful in the treatment of HIV-infected children."

Researchers from the University of Benin in Nigeria (Anukam *et al.* 2008) investigated probiotics in the treatment of HIV/AIDS in women. Yogurt with *Lactobacillus delbruekii* subsp. *bulgaricus, Streptococcus thermophilus, Lactobacillus rhamnosus* GR-1 and *L. reuteri* RC-14 was given to 24 HIV/AIDS adult female patients. Prior to treatment, they exhibited moderate diarrhea and CD4 counts over 200. They were not receiving antiretrovirals or other dietary supplements for 15 days prior to treatment. A placebo of conventional (unsupplemented) yogurt was used. The probiotic yogurt group was measured in the beginning, at 15 days and at 30 days. Average CD4 cell counts remained the same or increased in 11 of 12 supplemented probiotic subjects, compared with only 3 of 12 among the placebo group. Diarrhea, flatulence, and nausea were resolved in 12 of 12 probiotic patients within 2 days, versus 2 of 12 in the placebo group. The researchers concluded that this study, "suggests that perhaps a simple fermented food can provide some relief in the management of the AIDS epidemic in Africa."

Researchers from Yale University's School of Nursing (Williams *et al.* 2001) studied 164 HIV women with vaginal candidiasis. They were given either weekly vaginal applications of placebo, *Lactobacillus acidophilus* or clotrimazole for 21 months. Those using the probiotics experienced a significant reduction of episodes—similar to the results of the antifungal ointment clotrimazole.

Autoimmune/Inflammatory Diseases

In some ways, this section overlaps with some of the other topics because many diseases are described as autoimmune. Nevertheless, probiotics interact with the immune system in ways that help identify rouge cells more accurately. They do this by stimulating the immune factors appropriate to a particular type of problem. They also help to eliminate the possibility that these cells come under attack in the first place.

Researchers from China's Westchina Hospital and Sichuan University (Bai *et al.* 2006) took colonic biopsies from active ulcerative colitis patients. They were co-cultured for 24 hours with *Bifidobacterium longum*. Tumor necrosis factor (TNF)-alpha and interleukin (IL)-8 were lower than colitis patient samples cultured without *B. longum*. The number of lamina propria mononuclear cells (LPMC) with nuclear factor-kappa B (NF-kappaB) P65 positive among co-cultured tissues was also significantly less in the *B. longum* group. The researchers concluded that, "probiotics could inhibit NF-kappaB activation in LPMC and downlammatory cytokine secretion from inflamed tissues cerative colitis."

al researchers at the Università dell'Aquila in Italy (De Simone *et al.* 1992) gave *Bifidobacterium bifidum* and *Lactobacillus acidophilus* or placebo to 25 elderly persons for 28 days. After treatment, inflammatory factors among the subjects showed a significant reduction in colonic inflammation, without any altering of T-cells, B-cells and leu7 cells within the digestive system. B-cell activity within the intestinal peripheral bloodstream increased in the probiotic group. The researchers concluded that, "the overall results suggest that the regular administration of *B. bifidum* and *L. acidophilus* leads to a modulation of the immunological and inflammatory response in elderly subjects."

Healthy elderly volunteers were given either lactitol with a placebo or lactitol (a milk sugar-alcohol) plus *Lactobacillus acidophilus*. The group given the probiotics showed a modification of inflammatory markers (prostaglandin-1 and IgA); and produced levels of *Bifidobacterium* in the stool typical for younger persons with stronger immune systems (Ouwehand *et al.* 2009).

Scientists from the University of Helsinki (Kekkonen *et al.* 2008) measured lipids and inflammation markers before and after three weeks of treatment of *Lactobacillus rhamnosus* GG on 26 healthy adults. After three weeks, the probiotic decreased levels of inflammatory fatty acids lysophosphatidylcholines, sphingomyelins, and several glycerophosphatidylcholines. Meanwhile pro-inflammatory triglycerides decreased, and inflammatory markers TNF-alpha and CRP also decreased after the probiotic treatment.

Japanese scientists (Matsumoto and Benno 2006) found that acute inflammation was inhibited by the consumption of *Bifidobacterium lactis* LKM512 yogurt. Tumor necrosis factor (TNF)-alpha production was modulated, and inflammatory cytokines produced by macrophages were modulated—consistent with a reduction of inflammation.

Researchers from Japan's Osaka University Graduate School of Medicine (Shimizu *et al.* 2009) studied 58 patients with severe systemic inflammatory response syndrome (SIRS), and C-reactive protein (CRP) levels greater than 10 mg/dl. The patients received a placebo or a combination of *Bifidobacterium breve*, *Lactobacillus casei*, and GOS (prebiotic). Instances of enteritis, pneumonia, and bacteremia were significantly lower among the probiotic group compared to the placebo group. The probiotics significantly reduced complications in the SIRS patients.

University of Helsinki scientists (Kekkonen *et al.* 2008) also studied the possible anti-inflammatory effects of probiotics with 62 volunteers who received either a placebo or a milk-drink with either *Lactobacillus rhamnosus* GG, *Bifidobacterium animalis* subsp. *lactis*, or *Propionibacterium freudenreichii* subsp. *shermanii* JS. Fecal, venous blood and saliva samples were taken before, during and at the end of the trial period. Serum hsCRP levels were reduced in the all the probiotic groups. TNF-alpha from peripheral blood mononuclear cells was significantly lower in the *L. rhamnosus* LGG compared to the placebo group. IL-2 from peripheral blood mononuclear cells (PBMCs) was significantly lower in the *B. animalis* group compared to the placebo group. The researchers concluded that, "probiotic bacteria have strain-specific anti-inflammatory effects..."

Viruses: Colds, Influenza and Herpes

The immunostimulatory effects of probiotics have also been observed among some of the most frequent ailments known to humankind, including rhinovirus (colds), influenza virus (flu) and rotavirus (intestinal infections).

Viral influenza is now an important topic among medical experts, with the advent of the H1N1 swine flu epidemic that is threatening millions of people. While some have quoted statistics that from 25,000 to 35,000 people die each year of influenza, upon closer examination, well over 90% of those actually are elderly persons who die of pneumonia. Whether the flu or pneumonia is the official cause of death, the reason for these deaths is an overburdened and weakened immune system, not necessarily the flu or pneumonia itself.

Furthermore, despite valiant efforts by so many researchers over many decades, the "cure for the common cold" still eludes modern medicine. For most immune systems, this virus is not such a problem, because we typically can get over a cold within a few days. However, for those who are immunosuppressed, a simple cold can easily turn into pneunomia and other respiratory infections. In fact, many elderly people die from infections that began with a simple cold or the flu as mentioned above.

We are now faced with more risk of virulent influenza and other infectious outbreaks due to transcontinental flights and world travelers. Can probiotics help stave off viral infections? More importantly, can probiotics fight dangerous influenza viruses like H1N1? The answer lies in the ability of probiotics to specifically stimulate the immune system.

Scientists (Baron 2009) gave *Bacillus coagulans* GBI-30, 6086 to 10 healthy middle-aged men and women in a capsule for 30 days. After the treatment period, they had significantly increased T-cell production of TNF-alpha in response to adenovirus and influenza A (H3N2) exposure.

German scientists (de Vrese *et al.* 2005) gave a placebo or *Lactobacillus gasseri, Bifidobacterium longum* and *B. bifidum* to 479 healthy adult volunteers for three months. Total symptom score, duration of cold illness, and fever duration were significantly lower among the probiotic group—shortening common cold episodes by about 2 days—with a score was 79.3 versus 102.5 points. The probiotic group had significantly higher levels of cytotoxic T-suppressor cells (CD8+) and higher activity among T helper cells (CD4+), along with reduced severity of symptoms.

Finnish medical researchers from the University of Turku (Rautava *et al.* 2009) conducted a clinical study to see if probiotics could reduce infection risk during infancy. Infants younger than two months of age were given formula supplemented with *Lactobacillus rhamnosus* GG and *Bifidobacterium lactis* Bb-12 or a placebo daily until they were 12 months of age. Incidence of infections was 22% among the probiotic infants and 50% among the placebo group. In addition, 28% of those receiving probiotics contracted recurrent respiratory infections, compared to 55% of the placebo group.

In research that began in the late 1950s, Dr. Don Weekes clinically administered a combination of *L. acidophilus* and *L. bulgaricus* to 180 patients with ulcers and/or herpes infections. After average treatment times of three days with four-times daily doses, 61 of 64 patients with herpes simplex labialis, 77 of 97 patients with mouth ulcers (aphthous stomatitis), 6 of 13 patients with dendrites ulcers, and 6 of 6 patients with genital herpes were either "cured" or "much improved" from the probiotic treatments (Trenev 1998; Weekes 1983; Weekes 1958).

Bulgarian researchers have also confirmed herpes simplex inhibition from species of lactobacilli (Dimitonova *et al.* 2007).

One hundred children from a slum of New Delhi between two and five years old were given either a probiotic curd with *Lactobacillus acidophilus* or a placebo for six months. The probiotic group had more growth, and had fewer incidences of colds, flu, diarrhea and fever than the placebo group (Saran *et al.* 2002).

Scientists from Finland's University of Tampere (Isolauri *et al.* 1995) studied the administration of *Lactobacillus casei* GG with oral rotavirus vaccines given to 2-5-month-old infants. Infants receiving the probiotic displayed an increased level of rotavirus-specific IgM secreting cells. The researchers concluded that, "these findings suggest that LGG has an immunostimulating effect on oral rotavirus vaccination."

Scientists from Taiwan's Buddhist Tzu Chi General Hospital (Lin *et al.* 2009) gave 1,062 children under the age of five a placebo or *L. rhamnosus*. The children given the probiotic had significantly lower rates of bacterial, viral and respiratory infections, along with increased T-cell activity.

Swedish researchers (Tubelius *et al.* 2005) gave 262 healthy employees at Sweden's TetraPak company either *L. reuteri* or placebo for 80 days. During the study, the placebo group's sick leave reporting was 26.4% compared to 10.6% among the *L. reuteri* group. The sick-day frequency was 0.9% among the placebo group and 0.4% among the *L. reuteri* group. Among 53 shift-workers, 33% in the placebo group reported being sick during the study period as compared to none in the *L. reuteri* group.

Lactobacillus casei DN-114001 was given to 360 elderly people for 3 weeks by Italian researchers (Turchet *et al.* 2003). The probiotic group suffered a 20% shorter duration of winter illnesses compared to the placebo group.

Scientists from Italy's University of Milan (Pregliasco *et al.* 2008) gave placebo or several combinations of *Lactobacillus plantarum*, *Lactobacillus rhamnosus*, and *Bifidobacterium lactis* together with prebiotics to healthy volunteers over three winter seasons (2003-2007). Acute respiratory infection episodes and upper respiratory tract infections were significantly lower among the probiotic groups. Severity of all illness episodes decreased significantly among probiotic groups, ranging from .73 days less to 1.12 days less in average duration compared to the placebo groups. The duration of upper respiratory infections ranged from 1.51 days less to 2.07 days less than the placebo groups. The probiotic groups also had an average of 1.25 to 1.4 days less flu illnesses than the placebo groups. There was also significantly less cold illnesses among the probiotics groups compared to the placebo groups.

Sleep

Some studies (*in vivo*) have indicated that certain probiotics stimulate the production of tryptophan (Desbonnet *et al.* 2008). Because serotonin levels and reception are modulated in probiotic-deficient IBS and other digestive disorders (Harris and Chang, 2006), probiotics may well modulate serotonin levels and/or reception as well. These indicate the possibility of mechanisms for what has been observed clinically: Probiotics tend to subtly calm the nerves and increase quality sleep.

Scientists from Japan's Osaka University Graduate School of Medicine (Yamamura *et al.* 2009) gave *Lactobacillus helveticus* fermented milk to 29 healthy elderly volunteers 60-81 years old. After two treatment periods of 3 weeks separated by 3-week washout period, the probiotic group had a significant sleep efficiency improvement and a reduction of wakening episodes compared to the placebo group. There was also a small improvement in general health perception among the probiotic group.

Diabetes (Glucose Control)

Scientists from Finland's University of Turku Department of Biochemistry and Food Chemistry (Laitinen *et al.* 2009) studied the effects of probiotics on glucose metabolism in healthy pregnant women. Two hundred and fifty-six women in the first trimester of pregnancy were given either a placebo or a combination of *Lactobacillus rhamnosus* GG and *Bifidobacterium lactis* Bb12. Blood glucose concentrations were least among the probiotics group during their pregnancy period and through the 12 months' postpartum period.

Respiratory Infections

There is sufficient evidence that pathogenic bacteria such as *Staphylococcus aureus, Streptococcus pneumoniae* and *Heomonphilus influenzae* can infect the lungs. Little research seems to have been done to confirm whether or not the lungs also harbor probiotic bacteria, however. Research has confirmed that probiotic bacteria inhabit the nasal cavity, the mouth and the throat. Research has also confirmed that both ingested probiotics and probiotic sprays reduce lung infections. Probiotics in the lungs does not seem so radical: Certainly not as radical as the evidence showing probiotics from the intestinal tract can somehow inhibit bacteria in the lungs and nasal cavity.

In a study also mentioned earlier, scientists from the Swiss National Accident Insurance Institute (Glück and Gebbers 2003) gave 209 human volunteers either a conventional yogurt or a combination of *Lactobacillus* GG (ATCC 53103), *Bifidobacterium* sp. B420, *Lactobacillus acidophilus* 145, and *Streptococcus thermophilus* every day for 3 weeks. Nasal microbial flora was measured at the beginning, at day 21 and at day 28 (a week after). Significant pathogenic bacteria were found in most of the volunteers' nasal cavities at the beginning of the study. The consumption of the probiotic-enhanced milk led to a 19% reduction of pathogenic bacteria in the nasal cavity. The researchers concluded that, "The results indicate a [possible] linkage of the lymphoid tissue between the gut and the upper respiratory tract."

Scientists from Barcelona (Cobo Sanz *et al.* 2006) gave 251 children aged 3 to 12 years milk either with or without *Lactobacillus casei* for 20 weeks. The probiotic group of children experienced significantly less low respiratory tract infections, bronchitis and/or pneumonia (32% vs. 49%). The probiotic children also had a reduction in the duration of fatigue (3% vs. 13%). There was also a difference in the duration of sicknesses among the probiotic children compared to the placebo group.

French scientists (Forestier *et al.* 2008) assessed whether ventilator-associated pneumonia in intensive care units could be prevented or lessened by the use of probiotics. The 17-bed intensive care unit at the Clermont-Ferrand Teaching Hospital was used to test 208 patients with an intensive care unit stay of more than 48 hours. Patients were fed a placebo or *Lactobacillus rhamnosus* through a nasogastric feeding twice daily from their third day in the unit until discharge. Infective *Pseudomonas aeruginosa* cultures were measured at admission, once a week, and upon discharge. Bacteriological tests of the respiratory tract also were done to determine patient infections. The study results indicated that *P. aeruginosa* respiratory colonization and/or infection was significantly reduced among the probiotic group. Ventilator-associated pneumonia by *P. aeruginosa* in the probiotic group ws reduced by more than 50% compared to the placebo group.

Researchers from the University of Arkansas' Medical School (Wheeler *et al.* 1997) studied 15 asthmatic adults in two 1-month crossover periods with placebo or yogurt containing *L. acidophilus*. The probiotic consumption increased immune system interferon gamma and decreased eosinophilia levels.

Greek scientists from the Faculty of Medicine of the University of Thessaloniki (Kotzampassi *et al.* 2006) gave a placebo or probiotic combination to 65 elderly critically ill, mechanically ventilated, multiple trauma patients for 15 days. The combination consisted of *Pediococcus pentosaceus* 5-33:3, *Leuconostoc mesenteroides* 32-77:1, *L. paracasei* subsp. *paracasei* 19; and *L. plantarum* 2,362; and inulin, oat bran, pectin and resistant starch as prebiotics. The probiotic patients had significantly lower levels of infection, sepsis and death than did the placebo group. Number of days in the ICU and number of days under ventilation were significantly reduced compared to the placebo group. The researchers concluded that: "The administration of this synbiotic formula in critically ill, mechanically ventilated, multiple trauma patients seems to exert beneficial effects in respect to infection and sepsis rates and to improve the patient's response, thus reducing the duration of ventilatory support and intensive care treatment."

Scientists from the University of Buenos Aires (Río *et al.* 2002) studied the incidence and severity of respiratory tract infections. Fifty-eight children from 6 to 24 months old, normal or undernourished according to height-weight indexes, took either a placebo or a combination of live *Lactobacillus acidophilus* and *Lactobacillus casei* probiotics. Their episodes were classified as pneumonia, bronchitis, or recurrent obstructive bronchitis and upper respiratory tract infection. Total episodes in the probiotic group were 34, and 69 occurred in the placebo group. The probiotic combination significantly suppressed pneumonia and bronchitis in both the normal and undernourished probiotic groups.

Rebuilding the Immune System

For many of us in the modern industrialized world, we have overloaded and burdened our immune systems to the point where we are suffering from constant inflammation, recurrent infection, allergies or autoimmunity. Probiotics have been shown to significantly help these situations. Probiotics are nature's smart army corps of engineers. They will help rebuild cellular functions, immune cell function, and help stimulate better immune system responses.

Many studies have illustrated these effects. Furthermore, some of the research has confirmed that somehow, probiotics are able to stimulate the effects of vaccines. How are they able to do that? Remember that probiotics are living organisms that can become aware of a pathogen entering the body. Then they can assist the immune system by stimulating specific immune responses. In the case of a vaccine, the vaccine is a small quantity of the pathogen itself, which stimulates the immune system to develop strategies to attack and rid the body of that pathogen should it invade the body later. Because probiotics help identify and stimulate immune responses, researchers have found that vaccination is often more productive when it is done concurrent to probiotic supplementation.

In a German study (de Vrese *et al.* 2005), 64 volunteers took either probiotics (*Lactobacillus rhamnosus* GG or *Lactobacillus acidophilus* CRL431) or placebo for five weeks. During the second week of treatment, the volunteers were given oral vaccinations against poliovirus 1, 2 and 4. As reported in other research, polio vaccination—even as documented by Dr. Salk—has caused on occasion the contraction of polio. Poliovirus factors—evident from poliovirus neutralizing antibody titers—increased significantly with probiotic treatment in this study. Increased vaccination response with probiotics ranged from two- to four-times higher. Furthermore, serum levels of *poliovirus-specific* IgA and IgG antibodies were significantly increased in the probiotic group. The researchers concluded that, "Probiotics induce an immunologic response that may provide enhanced systemic protection of cells from virus infections by increasing production of virus neutralizing antibodies."

Researchers from France's Université de Picardie (Mullié *et al.* 2004) gave 30 infants aged zero to four months poliovirus vaccinations along with a formula with *B. longum* and *B. infantis* or a placebo. In the probiotic group, antipoliovirus IgA responses significantly increased among the probiotic group versus the placebo group that received the vaccinations without probiotics. Antibody titers correlated with bifidobacteria levels, especially with *B. longum/B. infantis* and *B. breve* supplementation doses. The researchers were puzzled by the mechanism, adding, "Whether this effect on the immune system is achieved through the bifidogenic effect of the formula (mainly through *B. longum/B. infantis* and *B. breve* stimulation) or directly linked to compounds (i.e. peptides) produced by milk fermentation remains to be investigated."

Scientists from Finland's University of Turku (Fang *et al.* 2000) gave *Lactobacillus* GG, *Lactococcus lactis* or placebo to 30 healthy volunteers for 7 days. On the first, third and fifth days, a *Salmonella typhi* Ty21 oral vaccine was given to each volunteer to mimic enteropathogenic infection. A greater increase in specific IgA was observed among the *Lactobacillus* GG group. Among the *L. lactis* group, significantly higher CR3 receptor expression on neutrophils was observed compared to the placebo or *Lactobacillus* GG groups. The researchers concluded that: "the immunomodulatory effect of probiotics is strain-dependent."

Scientists from Finland's University of Tampere (Isolauri *et al.* 1995) studied the administration of *Lactobacillus* GG with oral rotavirus vaccines given to 2-5-month-old infants. Infants receiving the probiotic displayed an increased level of rotavirus-specific IgM secreting cells. The researchers concluded that, "these findings suggest that LGG has an immunostimulating effect on oral rotavirus vaccination."

Rebuilding the immune system with probiotics will return to the system the most vital part of preventing opportunistic infections: acquired immunity.

Japanese scientists (Hirose *et al.* 2006) gave *Lactobacillus plantarum* strain L-137 or placebo to 60 healthy men and women, average age 56, for twelve weeks. Increased Con A-induced proliferation (acquired immunity), increases in IL-4 production by CD4+ T-cells, and a more balanced Th1:Th2 ratio was seen in the probiotic group. Quality of life criteria were also higher among the probiotic group.

Researchers from Britain's Scarborough Hospital (McNaught *et al.* 2005) gave a placebo or *Lactobacillus plantarum* 299v to 103 critically ill patients along with conventional therapy. On day 15, the probiotic group had significantly lower serum IL-6 levels compared to the control group.

Researchers from the Department of Immunology at Japan's Juntendo University School of Medicine (Takeda *et al.* 2006) gave a placebo or *Lactobacillus casei* Shirota to 9 healthy middle-aged adults and 10 elderly adults daily for three weeks. After three weeks of supplementation, *L. casei* significantly increased natural killer cell activity among the volunteers, especially among those who had low NK-cell activity before probiotic supplementation.

Researchers from the University of Vienna (Meyer *et al.* 2007) gave healthy women yogurt with starters *Lactobacillus bulgaricus* and *Streptococcus thermophilus*, with or without *Lactobacillus casei*. After two weeks, both yogurt groups had significantly increased blood levels of tumor necrosis factor-alpha (TNF-a): by 24% with the regular yogurt and by 63% with the *L. casei* yogurt. They also observed significantly higher levels of cytokines interleukin (IL)-1beta (by 40%) and interferon gamma (by 108%). In addition, IL-

10 decreased during *L. casei*-enhanced yogurt treatment, but then significantly increased after the yogurt treatment was stopped (by 129%).

French scientists (Paineau *et al.* 2008) gave 83 healthy volunteers a placebo or seven probiotic strains, and tested their resulting antibody levels and immune response rates. IgG levels increased in the *Bifidobacterium lactis* Bl-04 and *Lactobacillus acidophilus* La-14 groups, and increased serum immunoglobulin levels resulted from in six of the seven probiotic strains.

Researchers from the Department of Neurology and Geriatrics at Japan's Kagoshima University Graduate School of Medical and Dental Sciences (Matsuzaki *et al.* 2005) studied *Lactobacillus casei* Shirota as a treatment of HTLV-1 associated myelopathy/tropical spastic paraparesis. Ten HTLV-1 patients with myelopathy/tropical spastic paraparesis were given either a placebo or *Lactobacillus casei* Shirota fermented in milk for four weeks. NK-cell activity significantly increased. Spasticity—gauged by a modified Ashworth Scale—significantly decreased. Other urinary components indicating enhanced immunity were also seen following the probiotic treatment.

Researchers from Finland's University of Turku (Ouwehand *et al.* 2008) gave a placebo, *Bifidobacterium longum*, or *Bifidobacterium lactis* Bb-12 to 55 institutionalized elderly subjects for 6 months. The probiotic groups had modulated pro-inflammatory cytokine TNF-alpha and cytokine IL-10 levels compared with the placebo group.

Scientists from Spain's University of Navarra (Parra *et al.* 2004) investigated the effects of fermented milk with *Lactobacillus casei* DN114001 on 45 healthy volunteers, ages 51-58. The probiotic group showed increased oxidative burst capacity among monocytes, and increased NK-cell tumor suppression activity. The researchers concluded that *L. casei* can have "a positive effect in modulating the innate immune defense in healthy-middle-age people."

Nutritional Deficiencies

As discussed earlier, probiotics produce a number of nutrients needed by the body, including various B vitamins and vitamin K. The research confirms this:

Egyptian scientists (Mohammad *et al.* 2006) gave a large group of 11-year old children probiotic yogurt for 42 days. Prior to the study, 33.3% of the children presented with vitamin B12 deficiency and one-fifth were deficient in folate. Daily consumption of the probiotic yogurt significantly improved plasma levels of vitamin B12 and folate compared to before probiotic supplementation. The probiotic yogurt also caused a significant reduction in anemia among the children.

Researchers from Chile's Universidad de Antofagasta (Silva *et al.* 2008) gave 190 iron-deficient children from 2-5 years old either an iron-fortified probiotic drink with *Lactobacillus acidophilus* or an iron-fortified drink without probiotics for 101 days. The children who drank the probiotic drink had higher levels of red blood cells and a better balance between iron levels and hemoglobin than did the control group.

Researchers from the Department of Nutritional Sciences at the University of Vienna (Fabian *et al.* 2008) determined in a study of 33 young healthy women that eating 200 grams of yogurt a day increased blood and urine levels of thiamine (vitamin B1) and riboflavin (B2).

Interestingly, prior to the development of the 75Se-selenofolate radioassay, probiotic *L. casei* activity was used to measure folate levels (McGuire 1988).

Researchers from the Ramathibodi Hospital and Mahidol University in Thailand (Nopchinda *et al.* 2002) gave 148 children aged 6-36 months a placebo, *Bifidobacteria* Bb12, or a combination of Bb12 and *Streptococcus thermophilus* for six months. After the treatment period, the probiotic formula children showed greater growth than did the placebo group.

Researchers from Helsinki University (Narva *et al.* 2004) gave milk fermented with *Lactobacillus helveticus*-fermented milk or placebo milk to 20 postmenopausal women with an average age of 65. Juice was also tested to eliminate the possibility of the effects of milk tripeptides. The *L. helveticus* group significantly increased levels of elemental serum calcium and lower levels of parathyroid hormone (a common marker for bone calcium turnover). The researchers concluded that, "Fermentation of milk with *Lactobacillus helveticus* had a positive acute effect on calcium metabolism."

Though this study does not specifically confirm this, it is logical to assume that the decreased levels of parathyroid hormone and the increased serum calcium resulting from probiotic supplementation would also have a positive benefit upon the incidence of osteoporosis among probiotic supplement users.

Summary of Probiotic Mechanisms

We have seen a lot of research on the effects of probiotics. Let's summarize some of the basic functions, mechanisms and effects probiotics have shown among human clinical studies:

Allergies	reduce Th1/ Th2 ratio; decrease Th2 levels; lower TGF-beta2; increase IgE
Anorexia nervosa	increase appetite; increase assimilation; increase lymphocytes
Antibiotics	produce antibiotic and antifungal substances (such as acidophillin and bifidin) that repel or kill pathogenic bacteria, adjusting to pathogen and resistance
B-cells	modulate and redirect B-cell activity
Bile	break down bile acids
Biochemicals	secrete lactic acids, lactoperoxidases, formic acids, lipopolysaccharides, peptidoglycans, superantigens and others to manage pH and repel pathogens.

Bladder cancer	reduce recurrent bladder cancer incidence and inhibit new tumors
Blood pressure	reduce hypertension; inhibit ACE
Calcium	increase serum calcium; decrease parathyroid hormone
Cancer (general)	reduce mutagenicity; increase natural killer tumoricidal activity; increase survival rates
Candida overgrowth	control populations; reduce overgrowths
CD cell orientation	modulate and direct particular CD cells depending upon condition, including CD56, CD8, CD4, CD25, CD69, CD2, others
Cell degeneration	slow cellular degeneration and associated diseases among elderly persons
Colds and Influenza	reduce infection frequency; reduce infection duration; reduce symptoms; prevent complications; decrease worker sick days
Colic	reduce crying time; decrease infection; increase stool frequency; decrease bloating and indigestion
Colon cancer	reduce recurrence; increase survival rates; reduce beta-glucosidase; inhibit cell abnormality and mutation; increase IL-2
Constipation	increase bowel movement frequency; ease colon and impacted feces
Control pathogens	compete with pathogenic organisms for nutrients, thus checking their growth
C-reactive protein	reduce levels in blood
Cytokines	stimulate the body's production of various cytokines, including IL-6, IL-3, IL-5, TNF alpha, and interferon
Dental caries	reduce and control cavity-causing bacteria
Digestion	reduce gas, nausea and stress-related gastro-intestinal digestive difficulty
Digestive difficulty	secrete digestive enzymes; help break down nutrients from fats; proteins and other foods
Diverticulosis	reduce polyps and strengthen intestinal wall mucosa

Ear infections	hasten otitis media healing response; prevent infections
EFAs	manufacture essential fatty acids, including important short-chained FAs, and help body assimilate EFAs
Fiber digestion	aid in soluble fiber fermentation, yielding fatty acids and energy
Food poisoning	increase resistance to food poisoning; battle and remove pathogenic organisms; reduce diarrhea and other symptoms
Glucose metabolism	improve glucose control
Gum disease	reduce gum infections; deplete gingivitis
H. pylori	reduce *H. pylori* infections; reduce ulcers
HIV/AIDS	stimulate immune system; reduce symptoms; reduce co-infections; increase survival rates
Hormones	balance and stimulate hormone production
Hydrogen peroxide	manufacture H2O2 - oxygenating/antiseptic
IBS	decrease bloating, pain, cramping
Immunoglobulins	modulate IgA, IgG, IgE, IgM to weakness
Inflammation	modify prostaglandins (E1, E2), IFN-gamma, reduce CRP; modulate TNF-alpha; increase IgA; slow inflammatory response as needed
Intestinal Permeability	protect against IIPS; block penetration of toxins; work cooperatively with villi and microvilli; attach to mucosa; improve barrier function
Intestine walls	protect walls of intestines against toxin exposure and colonization of pathogens
Iron absorption	increase iron assimilation; increase hemoglobin count
Keratoconjunctivitis	decrease burning, itching and dry eyes
Kidney stones	reduce urine oxalates; reduce blood oxalates
Lipids/Cholesterol	reduce LDL, triglycerides and total cholesterol; increase HDL
Liver	stimulate liver cells (hepatocytes); stimulate liver function; reduce cirrhosis symptoms; reduce liver enzymes

Liver cancer	stimulate immune response; decrease infection and complications after surgery
Lung cancer	increase survival rates; reduce chest pain and other symptoms
Mental state	improve mood; stimulate positive mood hormones like serotonin and tryptophan
Milk digestion	aid dairy digestion for lactose-intolerant people; produce lactase
Monocytes	increase oxidative burst capacity
Mucosa	coat intestines, stomach, oral, nasal and vagina mucosa, providing protective barrier
NF-kappaB	modulate activity to condition
NK-cells	stimulate natural killer cell activity
Nutrition	manufacture biotin, thiamin (B1), riboflavin (B2), niacin (B3), pantothenic acid (B5), pyridoxine (B6), cobalamine (B12), folic acid, vitamin A and/or vitamin K; aid in assimilation of proteins, fats and minerals
Pancreatitis	reduce pancreas infection (sepsis); reduce necrosis; speed healing
pH control	produce a number of other acids and biochemicals, modulating pH (see biochemicals)
Phagocytes	increase phagocytic activity as needed
Phytonutrients	convert to bioavailable nutrient forms
Premature births and Low birth weights	speed growth; reduce infection; improve immune response; increase nutrition
Protein assimilation	break down amino acid content; inhibit assimilation of allergic polypeptides
Respiratory infections	inhibit pneumonia; reduce duration of infection; inhibit bronchitis; inhibit tonsillitis
Rotavirus infections	speed healing times; prevent infection; ease abdominal pain; eradicate infective agents
Spleen	stimulate spleen activity
Stomach cancer	inhibit tumors; reduce *H. pylori* overgrowths
T-cells	modulate T-cell activity to condition
Th1 - Th2	decrease Th2 activity; increase Th1 (increases healing and decreases allergic response)

Thymus	increase thymus size and activity
Toxins	break down toxins; inhibit assimilation of heavy metals, chemicals, and endotoxins
Ulcers	control *H. pylori*; speed healing; improve mucusa; moderate acids; reduce pain
Vaccination	increase vaccine effectiveness
Vaginosis/Vaginitis	reduce infection; re-establish healthy pH; reduce odor

This summary of primarily randomized, double-blinded, and placebo-controlled human clinical research is by no means a complete list of all the probiotic effects that have been found by researchers. Furthermore, medical scientists have only chosen a small portion of probiotics' possible health benefits for controlled human research. The effects shown in these studies illustrate a variety of other possible benefits for specific infections and diseases. As we can see from probiotics' ability to specifically stimulate the immune system, there are many other possible applications for probiotics in medicine. The research has only begun.

Meet Your Probiotics

As mentioned previously, there are trillions of bacteria in the body, and well over 400 different species inhabiting the mouth, nasal cavity, throat, lungs, stomach, intestines, colon, anus, vagina and other nooks and crannies of the body. Most of us go about our days oblivious to these tiny creatures keeping our bodies healthy from within. Let's meet some of these friendly creatures:

Species and Strains

The two most important groups of friendly bacteria are lactobacilli and bifidobacteria. These two genera, *Lactobacillus* and *Bifidobacterium* are only two of many genera that inhabit the body. Many others, such as *Eubacterium, Fusobacterium, Peptococaceae, Rheumanococcus* and *Streptococcus,* also cooperate within the body's cavities. These genus names differentiate the organisms by their cell qualities as well as activities. A further differentiation is the species name, which follows the genus. The species name further describes a particular organism. Within each species, however, there can be numerous subspecies.

Still within the species and subspecies can be different strains. A strain may be identified by its distinctive activities, effects, cell shape or other charcteristics. A strain may also be distinguished by its culture medium—in other words, a different habitat.

Large genetic differences can exist between different strains of the same probiotic bacteria species. Various *L. acidophilus* strains can differ up to 20% genetically, for example. In fact, some strains may not grow well in some people, while they might colonize prolifically in others.

Note that there are numerous probiotic subspecies strains that have been either isolated from different substrates or otherwise modified by scientists and commercial entities. There is evidence that some of these strains may be more vigorous than other strains of that species. However, conclusive evidence that these strains are necessarily more effective than every other strain of the same species has not been accomplished. Rigorous controlled, randomized and crossover studies would likely need to be performed to know this for certain. It may well be that what might make one strain stronger than another is not necessarily the strain, but the special fermentation medium in which the strain was cultured. A unique culture is likely to produce unique characteristics among any strain of the same species.

We certainly know that there is an economic incentive in developing and even patenting a strain by commercial concerns. Like pharmaceuticals, strain patents allow the patent-holder to exclusively produce and sell that particular strain for a period of time, while advertising with the research that has been performed on that strain.

This is not such a bad thing, however. It has enabled commercial interests to fund research on probiotics—which has benefited all of us. We are appreciative for the research, and even have no issue in buying their products with these possibly stronger strains. They also do not offer any significant restrictions to others who want to utilize the basic species or subspecies strains, either. Their research and their intent to spread the use of probiotics are commendable, and good for all of us.

In the final chart in the previous chapter, we summarized the human research by species without regard to strain. Keep in mind that some of these effects have been shown to occur with particular strains, or when certain strains were given in combination with other strains. In addition, some of the effects noted were with patients with specific ailments. These were mentioned in the earlier sections. Note that the particular effect (increasing a particular cytokine, for example) may well occur during a number of different ailments. This is part of the amazing benefit of probiotics: They will respond to individual needs because they are conscious organisms that seek the survival of their host, just as we should be seeking the survival of our mother earth.

Note also that the strain research focused on living human beings. There is also a huge library of animal research on probiotics, showing additional benefits not listed here. Animal studies, however, are inferior, especially for species- and strain-specific probiotics. Animal digestive tracts are typically quite different from human digestive tracts. Carnivorous animals, for example, will have short, fat digestive tracts, with lots of powerful enzymes that do not support many species of bacteria. Other animals, like grazing animals, have digestive tracts that are longer and more similar to ours, but these may host different strains at different populations than those hosted by humans. Thus determining for certain that certain probiotic species will benefit humans in certain ways is best accomplished through human clinical studies. This point has been confirmed by the finding of a variety of different species and strains of probiotics among different animals. While we know that many mammals do indeed host beneficial probiotics, we cannot necessarily apply those to human strain-specific probiotic effects.

Let's review the effects and characteristics of particular strains, based on the research reviewed earlier:

The Lactobacilli

Lactobacilli (*lactis* from Latin meaning "milk," and *bacillus* meaning "little rod") are primarily found in the small intestine. *Lactobacilli* will typically lower the pH of the intestine by converting long-chain saccharides (sugars) to lactic acid. This conversion process effectively inhibits pathogen growth and creates the appropriate acidic environment for lactobacilli to colonize.

Lactobacillus acidophilus

Lactobacillus acidophilus is by far the most familiar probiotic to most of us, and is also by far the most-studied probiotic species to date. They are one of the main residents of the human gut, although supplemented strains will still be transient. They are also found in the mouth and vagina. *L. acidophilus* grow best in warm (85-100 degrees F) and moist environments. Many are facultative anaerobic, meaning they can grow in oxygen-rich or oxygen-poor environments. *L. acidophilus* bacteria were first discovered by Llya Metchnikoff in the first decade of the twentieth century. Within a few years, *L. acidophilus* remedies were found in many venues, but they were poorly handled because many did not understand how easily probiotics would die outside of the intestines. Then in the late 1940s, scientists from the University of Nebraska began focused studies on *Lactobacillus acidophilus* to determine how to produce them, maintain them, and supply them as medicines.

Probably the most important benefit of *L. acidophilus* and the other probiotics is their ability to inhibit the growth of pathogenic bacteria, not only in the gut, but also throughout the body. *L. acidophilus* significantly controls and rids the body of *Candida albicans* overgrowth, which can invade various tissues of the body if unchecked. They also inhibit *Escherichia coli*, which can be fatal in large enough populations. They can also inhibit the growth of *Helicobacter pylori*—implicated in ulcers; *Salmonella*—a genus of deadly infectious bacteria; and *Shigella* and *Staphylococcus*—both potentially lethal infectious bacteria. It should be noted that *L. acidophilus'* ability to block these infectious agents will depend upon the size of the pathobiotic colonization and the size of the *L. acidophilus* colonies. *L. acidophilus* produces a variety of antibiotic substances, including acidolin, acidophillin, lactobacillin, lactocidin and others.

L. acidophilus and other probiotics will also lessen pharmaceutical antibiotic side effects; aid lactose absorption; help the absorption of various nutrients; help maintain the intestinal wall; help balance the pH of the upper intestinal tract; create a hostile environment for invading yeasts; and inhibit urinary tract and vaginal infections. Reports have shown the *L. acidophilus* species will specifically inhibit antibiotic-induced yeast infections.

The digestive effects of *L. acidophilus* include aiding the absorption of nutrients. In a study sponsored by India's National Institute of Nutrition (Saran *et al.* 2002), 100 malnourished two- to five-year old children were fed either 50ml fermented curd containing *L. acidophilus* or a placebo for six months. Significantly more weight gains (1.3 vs. .81 kg) and height gains (3.2 versus 1.7 cm) were noted from the group ingesting the probiotic compared to the control group, which ingested a similar curd without *L. acidophilus*. In addition, fewer cases of diarrhea (21 versus 35) and fever (30 versus 44) resulted. The authors of the study suggested that *L. acidophilus* aided in the repair of damaged intestinal epithelium due to gastrointestinal infection and lack of proper nutrition. They also suggested *L. acidophilus* assisted in promoting intestinal cellular repair.

L. acidophilus also produce several digestive enzymes including lactase, lipase and protease. Lactase is an enzyme that breaks down lactose. Several studies—as illustrated earlier—have shown that milk- or lactose-intolerant people are able to handle milk once they have established colonies of *L. acidophilus*. Lypase helps break down fatty foods, and protease helps break down protein foods.

The research indicates that under certain conditions, *L. acidophilus*:
- ❖ Lower LDL and total cholesterol
- ❖ Help digest milk
- ❖ Increase growth rates
- ❖ Reduce stress-induced GI problems
- ❖ Inhibit *E. coli*
- ❖ Reduce infection from rotavirus
- ❖ Reduce necrotizing enterocolitis

- ❖ Reduce intestinal permeability
- ❖ Control *H. pylori*
- ❖ Modulate PGE2 and IgA
- ❖ Reduce dyspepsia
- ❖ Modulate IgG
- ❖ Relieve and inhibit IBS and colitis
- ❖ Inhibit keratoconjunctivitis (in eye drops)
- ❖ Inhibit and control *Clostridium* spp.
- ❖ Inhibit *Bacteroides* spp.
- ❖ Inhibit and resolve acute diarrhea
- ❖ Reduce vaginosis and vaginitis
- ❖ Decrease triglycerides
- ❖ Increase appetite
- ❖ Increase growth in preterm infants
- ❖ Inhibit *Candida* spp. overgrowths
- ❖ Produce B vitamins and other nutrients
- ❖ Reduce anemia
- ❖ Increase vaccine efficiency
- ❖ Produce virus-specific antibodies
- ❖ Reduce allergic response
- ❖ Reduce urinary oxalate levels
- ❖ Inhibit antibiotic-related diarrhea
- ❖ Decrease allergic symptoms
- ❖ Inhibit upper respiratory infections
- ❖ Increase (good) HDL-cholesterol
- ❖ Inhibit tonsillitis
- ❖ Reduce blood pressure
- ❖ Inhibit viruses
- ❖ Increase leukocytes
- ❖ Increase calcium absorption

Lactobacillus helveticus

L. helveticus is a probiotic species popular in Switzerland. Latin *Helvetia* refers to the country of Switzerland. *L. helveticus* is often used as a cheese-making probiotic—especially for Swiss cheese—but also many other types of cheese. *L. helveticus* grow optimally between 102 and 122 degrees F. One of the reasons *L.*

helveticus are favored cheese starters is because they produce primarily lactic acid and not other metabolites which can make cheese taste bitter or sour. One of *L. helveticus'* more notable effects among the research has been their ability to reduce blood pressure.

The research has shown that under certain conditions, *L. helveticus*:
- ❖ Reduce blood pressure among hypertensive patients
- ❖ Produce ACE-inhibitor molecules
- ❖ Increase sleep quality and duration
- ❖ Increase general health perception
- ❖ Increase serum levels of calcium
- ❖ Decrease PTH (parathyroid hormone—marker for bone loss)
- ❖ Normalize gut colonization similar to breast-fed infants among formula-fed infants

Lactobacillus salivarius

Lactobacillus salivarius are typical residents of most humans— although supplemented versions will still be transients. They are also found in the intestines of other animals. *L. salivarius* will dwell in the mouth, the small intestines, the colon, and the vagina. They are hardy bacteria that can live in both oxygen and non-oxygen environments. *L. salivarius* is one of the few bacteria species that can also thrive in salty environments. They can also survive many antifungal medications.

This hardiness also means that *L. salivarius* can live in both the small intestines and the colon.

L. salivarius produce prolific amounts of lactic acid, which makes them hardy defenders of the teeth and gums. They also produce a number of antibiotics, and are speedy colonizers. Upon ingestion, they quickly combat pathogenic bacteria and create their territory. Because of their hardiness, they will readily take out massive numbers of pathogens immediately. *L. salivarius* are also known to be able to break apart complex proteins.

The research has shown that under certain conditions *Lactobacillus salivarius*:
- ❖ Inhibit mutans streptococci in the mouth
- ❖ Reduce dental carries
- ❖ Reduce gingivitis and periodontal disease
- ❖ Reduce mastitis
- ❖ Reduce risk of strep throat caused by *S. pyogenes*
- ❖ Reduce ulcerative colitis and IBS
- ❖ Inhibit *E. coli*
- ❖ Inhibit *Salmonella* spp.
- ❖ Inhibit *Candida albicans*

Lactobacillus casei

L. casei are transient bacteria within the human body. They are commonly used in a number of food applications and industrial applications. These include cheese-making, fermenting green olives, and fermenting milk products. *L. casei* is found naturally in raw milk and in colostrum—meaning they are residents of cow intestines. *L. casei* have been reported to reduce allergy symptoms and increase immune response. This seems to be accomplished by regulating the immune system's CHS, CD8 and T-cell responsiveness. However, this immune stimulation seems to be evident primarily among immunosuppressed patients (Guerin-Danan *et al.* 1998). This of course is another indication that probiotics uniquely respond to the host's particular condition. Some strains of *L. casei* are also very aggressive, and within a mixed probiotic supplement or food, they can dominate and even remove the other bacteria.

The research has shown that under certain conditions, *L. casei*:
- ❖ Inhibit pathogenic microbial infections
- ❖ Reduce occurrence, risk and symptoms of IBS
- ❖ Inhibit severe systemic inflammatory response syndrome
- ❖ Decrease C-reactive protein (CRP)
- ❖ Inhibit pneumonia
- ❖ Inhibit respiratory tract infections

- ❖ Inhibit bronchitis
- ❖ Maintain remission of diverticular disease
- ❖ Inhibit *H. pylori* (and ulcers)
- ❖ Reduce allergy symptoms
- ❖ Inhibit *Pseudomonas aeruginosa*
- ❖ Decrease milk intolerance
- ❖ Increase CD3+ and CD4+
- ❖ Increase phagocytic activity
- ❖ Support liver function
- ❖ Decrease risk of cirrhosis
- ❖ Decrease cytokine TNF-alpha
- ❖ Stimulate the immune system
- ❖ Inhibit and reduce diarrhea episodes
- ❖ Produce vitamins B1 and B2
- ❖ Prevent recurrence of bladder cancer
- ❖ Stimulate cytokine interleukin-1beta (IL-1b)
- ❖ Stimulate interferon-gamma
- ❖ Inhibit *Clostridium difficile*
- ❖ Reduce asthma symptoms
- ❖ Reduce constipation
- ❖ Decrease beta-glucuronidase (associated with colon cancer)
- ❖ Stimulate natural killer cell activity (NK-cells)
- ❖ Increase IgA levels
- ❖ Increase lymphocytes
- ❖ Decrease IL-6 (pro-inflammatory)
- ❖ Increase IL-12 (stimulates NK-cells)
- ❖ Reduce lower respiratory infections
- ❖ Inhibit *Candida* overgrowth
- ❖ Inhibit vaginosis
- ❖ Prevent colorectal tumor growth
- ❖ Restore NK-cell activity in smokers
- ❖ Stimulate the immune system among the elderly
- ❖ Increase oxygen burst activity of monocytes
- ❖ Increase CD56 lymphocytes
- ❖ Decrease rotavirus infections
- ❖ Decrease colds and influenza
- ❖ Reduce risk of bladder cancer

❖ Increase (good) HDL-cholesterol
❖ Decrease triglycerides
❖ Decrease blood pressure
❖ Inhibit viral infections
❖ Inhibit malignant pleural effusions secondary to lung cancer
❖ Reduce cervix tumors when used in combination radiation therapy
❖ Inhibit tumor growth of carcinomatous peritonitis/stomach cancer
❖ Break down nutrients for bioavailability

Lactobacillus rhamnosus

This species was previously thought to be a subspecies of *L. casei*. *L. rhamnosus* is a common ingredient in many yogurts and other commercial probiotic foods. *L. rhamnosus* have also been extensively studied over the years. Much of this research has centered around a particular strain, *L. rhamnosus* GG. *L. rhamnosus* GG have been shown in numerous studies to significantly stimulate the immune system and inhibit a variety of infections. This strain also has shown to have good intestinal wall adhesion properties. This is not to say, however, that non-GG strains will not perform similarly. In fact, studies with *L. rhamnosus* GR-1, *L. rhamnosus* 573/L, and *L. rhamnosus* LC705 strains have also showed positive results. The GG strain (LGG is trademarked by the Valio Ltd. Company in Finland) was patented in 1985 by two scientists, Dr. Sherwood Gorbach and Dr. Barry Goldin (hence the G&G). This patent and trademark, of course, gives these companies the incentive to fund expensive research to show the properties of this strain. Thanks to them, we have found that *Lactobacillus rhamnosus* (or the GG strain specifically) has a number of the health-promoting properties.

The research has shown that under certain conditions, *L. rhamnosus*:
❖ Inhibit a number of pathogenic microbial infections
❖ Improve glucose control
❖ Reduce risk of ear infections
❖ Reduce risk of respiratory infections

- ❖ Decrease beta-glucosidase
- ❖ Inhibit vaginosis
- ❖ Reduce eczema
- ❖ Reduce colds and flu
- ❖ Stimulate the immune system
- ❖ Increase IgA levels in mouth mucosa
- ❖ Increase IgA levels in mothers breast milk
- ❖ Inhibit *Pseudomonas aeruginosa* infections in respiratory tract
- ❖ Inhibit *Clostridium difficile*
- ❖ Increase immune response in HIV/AIDS patients
- ❖ Decrease symptoms of HIV/AIDS
- ❖ Inhibit rotavirus
- ❖ Inhibit enterobacteria
- ❖ Reduce IBS symptoms
- ❖ Decrease IL-12, IL-2+ and CD69+ T-cells in IBS
- ❖ Reduce constipation
- ❖ Inhibit vancomycin-resistant enterococci (antibiotic-resistant)
- ❖ Reduce the risk of colon cancer
- ❖ Modulate skin IgE sensitization
- ❖ Inhibit *H. pylori* (ulcer-causing)
- ❖ Reduce atopic dermatitis in children
- ❖ Increase Hib IgG levels in allergy-prone infants
- ❖ Reduce colic
- ❖ Stimulate infant growth
- ❖ Stimulate IgM, IgA and IgG levels
- ❖ Stabilize intestinal barrier function (decreased permeability)
- ❖ Increase INF-gamma
- ❖ Modulate IL-4
- ❖ Help prevent atopic eczema
- ❖ Reduce *Streptococcus mutans*
- ❖ Stimulate tumor killing activity among NK-cells
- ❖ Modulate IL-10 (anti-inflammatory)
- ❖ Reduce inflammation
- ❖ Reduce LDL-cholesterol levels

Lactobacillus reuteri

L. reuteri is a species found residing permanently in humans. As a result, most supplemented strains attach fairly well, though temporarily, and stimulate colony growth for resident *L. reuteri* strains. *L. reuteri* will colonize in the stomach, duodenum and ileum regions. *L. reuteri* will also significantly modulate the immune response of the gastrointestinal mucosal membranes. This means that *L. reuteri* are useful for many of the same digestive ailments that *L. acidophilus* are also effective for. *L. reuteri* also have several other effects, including the restoration of our oral cavity bacteria. They also produce a significant amount of antibiotic biochemicals.

The research has shown that under certain conditions, *L. reuteri*:
- Inhibit gingivitis
- Reduce pro-inflammatory cytokines
- Help re-establish the pH of the vagina
- Stimulate growth and feeding among preterm infants
- Inhibit and suppress *H. pylori*
- Decrease dyspepsia
- Increase CD3+ in HIV patients
- Reduce nausea
- Reduce flatulence
- Reduce diarrhea (rotavirus and non-rotavirus)
- Reduce TGF-beta2 in breast-feeding mothers (reduced risk of eczema)
- Reduce salivary *mutans streptococcus*
- Stimulate the immune system
- Reduce plaque on teeth
- Inhibit vaginal candidiasis
- Decrease symptoms of IBS
- Increase CD4+ and CD25 T-cells (in IBS)
- Decrease TNF-alpha (in IBS)
- Decrease IL-12 (in IBS)
- Reduce IgE eczema in infancy
- Reduce infant colic

❖ Restore vagina pH
❖ Reduce colds and influenza
❖ Stabilize intestinal barrier function (reducing intestinal permeability)
❖ Decrease atopic dermatitis

Lactobacillus plantarum

L. plantarum has been part of the human diet for thousands of years. They are active in cultures of sauerkraut, gherkin and olive brines. They are used to make sourdough bread, Nigerian ogi and fufu, kocha from Ethiopia, and sour mifen noodles from China, Korean kim chi and other traditional foods. *L. plantarum* are also found in dairy and cow dung.

L. plantarum is a hardy strain. The bacteria have been shown to survive all the way through the intestinal tract, into the stool. Temperature for optimal growth is 86-95 degrees F. *L. plantarum* are not permanent residents, however. When supplemented, they vigorously attack pathogenic bacteria, and create an environment hospitable for incubated resident strains to expand. *L. plantarum* also produce lysine, and a number of antibiotics including lactolin.

The research has shown that under certain conditions, *L. plantarum*:
❖ Reduce burn infections (topical)
❖ Increase burn healing
❖ Strengthen the immune system
❖ Help restore healthy liver enzymes (in mild alcohol-induced liver injury)
❖ Reduce frequency and severity of respiratory diseases during the cold and flu season
❖ Reduce intestinal permeability
❖ Inhibit various intestinal pathobiotics (such as *Clostridium difficile*)
❖ Reduce Th2 (inflammatory) levels and increase Th1/Th2 ratio
❖ Reduce inflammatory responses

❖ Reduce symptoms and aid healing of multiple traumas among injured patients
❖ Reduce fungal infections
❖ Reduce IBS symptoms
❖ Reduce pancreatic sepsis (infection)
❖ Reduce systolic blood pressure
❖ Reduce leptin levels
❖ Reduce interleukin-6 (IL-6) levels
❖ Reduce adhesion of vein endothelial cells by monocytes (risk of atherosclerosis)
❖ Reduce postoperative infection
❖ Reduce risk of pneumonia
❖ Reduce kidney oxalate levels
❖ Decrease flatulence
❖ Stimulate immunity in HIV children

Lactobacillus bulgaricus

We owe the *bulgaricus* name to Ilya Mechnikov, who named it after the Bulgarians—who used the bacteria to make the fermented milks that appeared related to their extreme longevity. In the 1960s and 1970s Russian researchers, notably Dr. Ivan Bogdanov and others, began focused research on first the secretions of *L. bulgaricus* and later on fragmented cell walls of the bacteria. Early studies indicated antitumor effects. As the research progressed into Russian clinical research and commercialization, it became obvious that *L. bulgaricus* cell fragments have a host of immune-stimulation benefits.

L. bulgaricus bacteria are transients that assist in *bifidobacteria* colony growth. They significantly stimulate the immune system and have been shown to have antitumor and anticancer effects. They also produce antibiotic and antiviral substances such as bulgarican and others. *L. bulgaricus* bacteria have been reported to have anti-herpes effects as well. *L. bulgaricus* require more heat to colonize than many probiotics—at 104-109 degrees F.

The research has shown that under certain conditions, *L. bulgaricus*:
- ❖ Reduce intestinal permeability
- ❖ Decrease IBS symptoms
- ❖ Help manage HIV symptoms
- ❖ Stimulate TNF-alpha
- ❖ Stimulate IL-1beta
- ❖ Decrease diarrhea (rotavirus and non-rotavirus)
- ❖ Decrease nausea
- ❖ Increase phagocytic activity
- ❖ Increase leukocyte levels
- ❖ Increase immune response
- ❖ Increase CD8+ levels
- ❖ Lower CD4+/CD8+ ratio (lower CD4+—associated with inflammation)
- ❖ Increase IFN-gamma
- ❖ Lower total cholesterol
- ❖ Lower LDL levels
- ❖ Lower triglycerides
- ❖ Inhibit viruses
- ❖ Reduce salivary mutans in the mouth
- ❖ Increase absorption of dairy (lactose)
- ❖ Increase white blood cell counts after chemotherapy
- ❖ Increase IgA specific to rotavirus (increased immunity against rotavirus)
- ❖ Reduce intestinal bacteria

Lactobacillus brevis

L. brevis are natural residents of cow intestines. They are therefore found in raw milk, colostrum, and cheese. They are transient in humans, but there is also the possibility that they are involved in early resident colonization and possibly even permanent residency among the human intestines.

The research has shown that under certain conditions, *L. brevis*:
- ❖ Reduce periodontal disease
- ❖ Reduce PGE2 levels
- ❖ Reduce IFN-gamma levels

❖ Reduce mouth ulcers
❖ Reduce urinary oxalate levels (kidney stones)
❖ Decrease *H. pylori* colonization

Other lactobacilli species showing benefits in clinical research include *Lactobacillus gasseri*, *Lactobacillus kefir*, *Lactobacillus delbrueckii*, *Lactobacillus jugurti* and others. These isolated, cultured and researched species are still only a few of the many probiotic species that exist inside and outside our bodies.

The Bifidobacteria

Bifidobacteria (*bifid* from Latin meaning "two parts") are primarily found in the colon. They also colonize (yes, they *colon*-ize) in great numbers, inhabiting large sections of the colon, primarily within the mucoid plaque that lies close to the intestinal wall. Here they work with the body to help process our waste matter and help break down remaining micronutrients from foods before they are excreted. Infants typically begin with *bifidobacteria infantis* colonies. With age, these colonies are joined by other species of bifidobacteria, including *Bifidobacterium longum* and *Bifidobacterium brevis* among others.

Bifidobacteria significantly outnumber lactobacilli in the intestines. Well over 90% of healthy colon bacteria will be bifidobacteria. Bidifobacteria are thus critical to the processing of bile and liver chemicals that circulate between the colon, liver and intestines. This pathway also provides a conduit for endotoxins from pathogens to enter the bloodstream. Having sufficient bifidobacteria is thus important for keeping the bloodstream clear of endotoxins. Healthy infants have a predominance of bifidobacteria, and healthy mother's breast milk will have large bifidobacteria counts. However, bifidobacteria numbers can be depleted over the years. Elderly people will often have drastically smaller counts of bifidobacteria—which is a contributing factor for early degeneration.

Some of the specific benefits of bifidobacteria include the manufacture of all-important B-vitamins; the inhibition of yeasts and nitrate-producing bacteria; the production of acids to balance pH; the lessening of antibiotic side effects; the prevention of toxin absorption; and the regulation of peristalsis. Let's discuss a few of the bifidobacteria species more specifically:

Bifidobacterium bifidum

These are normal residents in the human intestines, and by far the largest residents in terms of colonies. They are also sometimes inhabitants of healthy vaginas. Their greatest populations occur in the colon. They also inhabit the lower small intestinal tract. Breast milk typically contains large populations of *B. bifidum* along with other bifidobacteria. *B. bifidum* are highly competitive with yeasts such as *Candida albicans*. As a result, their populations may be decimated by large yeast overgrowths. This will also result in a number of endotoxins, including ammonia, being leached out of the colon into the bloodstream. As a result, *B. bifidum* populations are extremely important to the health of the liver, as has been illustrated in the research. They produce an array of antibiotics such as bifidin and various antimicrobial biochemicals such as formic acid. *B. bifidus* populations can also be severely damaged by the use of pharmaceutical antibiotics.

The research has shown that under certain conditions, *B. bifidum*:
- ❖ Reduce liver enzymes
- ❖ Increase cell regeneration in alcohol-induced liver injury
- ❖ Reduce death among very low birth weight infants
- ❖ Stimulate immunity in very low birth weight infants
- ❖ Increase TGF-beta (anti-inflammatory) levels
- ❖ Reduce allergies
- ❖ Stimulate the immune system among HIV-infected children
- ❖ Reduce *H. pylori* colonization

- ❖ Increase CD8+ T-cells as needed
- ❖ Establish infant microflora
- ❖ Inhibit *E. coli*
- ❖ Reduce intestinal bacteria infections
- ❖ Reduce acute diarrhea (rotavirus and non-rotavirus)

Bifidobacterium infantis

B. infantis are also normal residents of the human intestines—primarily among children. As implicated in the name, infants colonize a significant number of *B. infantis* in their early years. They will also colonize in the vagina, leading to the newborn's first exposure to protective probiotic bacteria (before the various pathogenic bacteria of the outside world get in). For this reason, it is important that pregnant mothers consider probiotic supplementation with *B. infantis*. *B. infantis* are largely anaerobic, and thrive within the darkest regions, where they can produce profuse quantities of acetic acid, lactic acid and formic acid to acidify the intestinal tract.

The research has shown that under certain conditions, *B. infantis*:
- ❖ Reduce acute diarrhea (rotavirus and non-rotavirus)
- ❖ Reduce or eliminate symptoms of IBS
- ❖ Reduce death among very low birth weight infants
- ❖ Increase immunity among very low birth weight infants
- ❖ Establish infant microflora
- ❖ Normalize Th1/Th2 ratio
- ❖ Reduce inflammatory allergic responses
- ❖ Normalize IL-10/IL-12 ratio
- ❖ Improve immune system efficiency
- ❖ Increase antipoliovirus IgA levels following vaccination
- ❖ Reduce urinary oxalate (kidney stones)

Bifidobacterium longum

B. longum are also normal inhabitants of the human digestive tract. They are one of the top four bifidobacteria inhabitants. Like *B. infantis*, they produce acetic, lactic and formic acid. Like other bifidobacteria, they resist the growth of pathogenic bacteria, and thus reduce the production of harmful nitrites and ammonia. *B. longum* also produce B vitamins. Breast milk contains significant *B. longum.* Latin *longus* means "long."

The research has shown that under certain conditions, *B. longum*:
- ❖ Reduce death among very low birth weight infants
- ❖ Reduce sickness among very low birth weight infants
- ❖ Reduce acute diarrhea (rotavirus and non-rotavirus)
- ❖ Reduce vomiting
- ❖ Reduce nausea
- ❖ Reduce ulcerative colitis
- ❖ Reduce or alleviate symptoms of IBS
- ❖ Stabilize intestinal barrier function (decreased permeability)
- ❖ Inhibit *H. pylori*
- ❖ Increase TGF-beta1 (anti-inflammatory) levels
- ❖ Decrease (inflammatory) TNF-alpha
- ❖ Decrease (inflammatory) IL-10 cytokines
- ❖ Reduce lactose-intolerance symptoms
- ❖ Reduce diarrhea
- ❖ Increase helper T-cells type2 (Th2)
- ❖ Increase IL-6
- ❖ Reduce Th1
- ❖ Reduce pro-inflammatory IL-12 and interferon
- ❖ Stimulate healing of liver in cirrhosis
- ❖ Reduce constipation
- ❖ Reduce hypersensitivity
- ❖ Reduce IBS symptoms
- ❖ Inhibit intestinal pathogenic bacteria
- ❖ Decrease prostate cancer risk
- ❖ Decrease itching, nasal blockage and rhinitis in allergies
- ❖ Reduce NF-kappaB
- ❖ Reduce IL-8 levels
- ❖ Reduce progression of chronic liver disease
- ❖ Reduce incidence and duration of common cold
- ❖ Increase antipoliovirus IgA levels following vaccination
- ❖ Reduce total cholesterol levels

- ❖ Increase HDL-cholesterol levels
- ❖ Increase absorption of dairy

Bifidobacterium animalis/B. lactis

B. animalis was previously thought to be distinct from B. lactis, but today they are considered the same species with B. lactis being a subspecies of B. animalis. B. lactis has also been described as Streptococcus lactis. They are transient bacteria typically present in raw milk. They are also used as starters for cheese, cottage cheese and buttermilk, and also found among certain plants.

The research has shown that under certain conditions, B. animalis:
- ❖ Reduce constipation
- ❖ Improve digestive comfort
- ❖ Decrease total cholesterol
- ❖ Increase blood glucose control
- ❖ Reduce risk of otitis media
- ❖ Reduce respiratory diseases (severity and frequency)
- ❖ Reduce colds and flu
- ❖ Strengthen the immune system
- ❖ Reduce salivary mutans in mouth
- ❖ Increase body weight among preterm infants
- ❖ Increase vaccination immune response
- ❖ Reduce CRP (inflammatory) levels
- ❖ Reduce TNF-alpha (inflammatory) levels
- ❖ Reduce acute diarrhea (rotavirus and non-rotavirus)
- ❖ Reduce IL-10 (inflammatory) levels
- ❖ Reduce TGF-beta1 (inflammatory) levels
- ❖ Reduce inflammatory responses
- ❖ Reduce CDE4+CD54(+) (inflammatory) cytokines
- ❖ Stimulate improvement in atopic dermatitis patients
- ❖ Reduce IBS symptoms
- ❖ Reduce diarrhea
- ❖ Normalize bowel movements
- ❖ Decrease intestinal permeability

❖ Reduce blood levels of interferon-gamma
❖ Stimulate IgA cells among milk-allergy infants
❖ Improve atopic dermatitis symptoms and sensitivity
❖ Inhibit *H. pylori*
❖ Increase HDL-cholesterol
❖ Reduce allergic inflammation
❖ Increase T-cell activity as needed
❖ Increase immunity among the elderly
❖ Increase tumoricidal activity
❖ Increase natural killer cell activity
❖ Reduce dental caries
❖ Increase absorption of dairy

Bifidobacterium breve

B. breve are also normal inhabitants of the human digestive tract—living mostly within the colon. They produce prolific acids, and also B vitamins. Like the other bifidobacteria, they also reduce ammonia-producing bacteria in the colon, aiding the health of the liver. Latin *brevis* means short.

The research has shown that under certain conditions, *B. breve*:
❖ Reduce severe systemic inflammatory response syndrome
❖ Increase resistance to respiratory infection
❖ Reduce TNF-alpha (inflammatory)
❖ Reduce IL-10 (inflammatory)
❖ Reduce TGF-beta1 (inflammatory)
❖ Reduce IBS symptoms
❖ Decrease beta-glucoronidase (colon tumor-causing)
❖ Inhibit *H. pylori*
❖ Increase antipoliovirus vaccination effectiveness
❖ Reduce acute diarrhea (rotavirus and non-rotavirus)
❖ Reduce allergy symptoms
❖ Increase growth weights among very low birth weight infants

Other Notable Probiotics

There are a variety of other bacteria that dwell peacefully and symbiotically in our guts, mouths and other areas. The list is growing longer, however, as we are continuing to find new beneficial species that either dwell as residents in our bodies or are able to reside temporarily as supplemental species.

Some of these are considered probiotic in practically any colony size. Some are pathogenic if they are allowed to overgrow their typical colony sizes. Like any population, once things get out of control, even the most beneficial species can produce negative effects. While these could also be referred to as eubiotics, their many beneficial effects from the research have been enough to earn the coveted "probiotics" title.

Streptococcus thermophilus

Streptococcus thermophilus are common participants in yogurt making. They are also used in cheese making, and are even sometimes found in pasteurized milk. They will colonize at higher temperatures, from 104-113 degrees F. This is significant because this bacterium readily produces lactase, which breaks down lactose. This is the only known streptococci that will do this. Like other supplemented probiotics, *S. thermophilus* are temporary microorganisms in the human body. Their colonies will typically inhabit the system for a week or two before exiting. During that time, however, they will help set up a healthy environment to support resident colony growth. Like other probiotics, *S. thermophilus* also produce a number of different antibiotic substances, including acids that deter the growth of pathogenic bacteria.

<u>The research has shown that under certain conditions, *S. thermophilus*</u>:
- ❖ Reduce acute diarrhea (rotavirus and non-rotavirus)
- ❖ Reduce intestinal permeability
- ❖ Inhibit *H. pylori*
- ❖ Help manage AIDS symptoms
- ❖ Increase lymphocytes among low-WBC patients
- ❖ Increase IL-1beta
- ❖ Decrease IL-10
- ❖ Increase tumor necrosis factor-alpha (TNF-a)
- ❖ Increase absorption of dairy
- ❖ Decrease symptoms of IBS
- ❖ Inhibit *Clostridium difficile*
- ❖ Increase immune function among the elderly
- ❖ Restore infant microflora similar to breast-fed infants
- ❖ Increase CD8+
- ❖ Increase IFN-gamma
- ❖ Reduce acute gastroenteritis (diarrhea)
- ❖ Reduce baby colic
- ❖ Reduce symptoms of atopic dermatitis
- ❖ Reduce nasal cavity infections
- ❖ Increase HDL-cholesterol
- ❖ Increase growth in preterm infants
- ❖ Reduce intestinal bacteria
- ❖ Reduce upper respiratory tract infections from *Staphylococcus aureus*, *Streptococcus pneumoniae*, beta-hemolytic streptococci, and *Haemophilus influenzae*
- ❖ Increase HDL cholesterol
- ❖ Reduce urine oxalates (kidney stones)
- ❖ Reduce salivary mutans streptococci in the mouth
- ❖ Reduce flare-ups of chronic pouchitis
- ❖ Reduce LDL-cholesterol in overweight subjects
- ❖ Reduce ulcerative colitis

Bacillus coagulans

Bacillus coagulans are endospore-forming bacteria that more closely resemble a soil-based organism. Nonetheless, *B. coagulans* can also be typical residents in the human digestive tract in controlled numbers. They were isolated in the 1930s, and named *Lactobacillus sporogenes*. Later scientists renamed the species into its current genus.

B. coagulans are considered friendly organisms in controlled numbers and have a propensity for aiding the human body and attacking invading organisms. The strain is known as one of the most immune-stimulating bacteria available. It has been shown in vitro to activate IgM—blood and lymph immunoglobulins associated with the body's first response for a number of infections; IgG—body fluid antibodies which respond to bacteria and viruses; and IgA antibody activity. *B. coagulans* bacteria are commonly used therapeutically throughout Germany, France and Israel to repel infection.

B. coagulans are spore-formers. This means they will multiply through the use of internally produced spores. These spores are surrounded by a tough exosporium or covering, making the spores resilient in harsh environments. This is a good thing in terms of survival through the stomach acids. At the same time, this endospore forming method of propagation contrasts that of most probiotics—simple binary fission and division. This means *B. coagulans* can be more resilient throughout their occupation in the body. Assuming they are eventually controlled by other probiotics, there should be no problem. However, left alone without a balance of other probiotic species…. well, this has not been well studied. Other notable endospore-forming bacteria include *Clostridium difficile*.

The research has shown that under certain conditions, *B. coagulans*:
- ❖ Reduce bloating in IBS
- ❖ Reduce abdominal pain in IBS
- ❖ Increase T-cell production of TNF-alpha in response to influenza A and adenovirus exposures

Enterococcus faecium

This species was formerly referred to as *Streptococcus faecium*. There are many strains of *E. faecium*, and they can range from being probiotics to pathogens. Probiotic versions are sometimes used to make cheeses, and they are also available in a number of supplement products as well. *E. faecium* are extremely hardy, and can handle extreme temperature and pH conditions. As a result, it is quite easy to get *E. faecium* through the stomach's acids.

The research has shown that under certain conditions, *E. faecium*:
- ❖ Decrease levels of sICAM-1 and CD54 (blood pressure adhesion) on monocytes
- ❖ Decrease CD11b (blood pressure adhesion) on lymphocytes
- ❖ Reduce blood vessel adhesion
- ❖ Reduce acute diarrhea
- ❖ Reduce beta-glucuronidase (associated with colon cancer)
- ❖ Increase superoxide and other antioxidant substances
- ❖ Increase IgG from peripheral blood mononuclear cells
- ❖ Increase myeloperoxidase and elastase in peripheral neutrophils
- ❖ Reduce total cholesterol
- ❖ Reduce LDL-cholesterol
- ❖ Decrease blood pressure
- ❖ Reduce endotoxin levels among cirrhosis patients
- ❖ Decrease abdominal pain and frequency of IBS symptoms

Saccharomyces boulardii

S. boulardii are yeasts (fungi). They render a variety of preventative and therapeutic benefits to the body planet. Yet should this or another yeast colony grow too large, they can quickly become a burden to the body due to their dietary needs (primarily refined sugars) and waste products. *S. boulardii* are known to enhance IgA—the antibody immunoglobulin focused on skin and mucosal membrane immunity. This is likely why this probiotic helps clear skin disorders. *S. boulardii* also help control diarrhea, and have been shown to be helpful in Crohn's Disease and irritable bowel issues. *S. boulardii* have been shown to be useful in combating cholera bacteria (*Vibrio cholerae*) as well.

<u>The research has shown that under certain conditions, *S. boulardii*:</u>

- ❖ Decrease infectious *Entameba histolytica* (intestinal)
- ❖ Inhibit *H. pylori*
- ❖ Decrease intestinal permeability
- ❖ Decrease diarrhea infections
- ❖ Stimulate T-cells as needed
- ❖ Decrease C-reactive protein
- ❖ Decrease beta-glucoronidase enzyme (associated with colon cancer)
- ❖ Inhibit *E. coli*
- ❖ Reduce ulcerative colitis
- ❖ Reduce symptoms of Crohn's disease
- ❖ Reduce *Clostridium difficile*
- ❖ Decrease parathyroid hormone—marker for bone loss

Soil-based Organisms

Soil-based organisms such as *Bacillus laterosporus*, *Bacillus sphaericus*, *Bacillus coagulins* (also described earlier), and *Bacillus subtilis* have become controversial in the discussion regarding probiotic supplementation. There has been a strong contingent among health proponents promoting soil-based organisms as probiotic supplements. It should be known, however, that these soil-based organisms are typically spore-formers. These are the same type of organisms that cause pathogenic bacteria growth. They also can grow at incredible speeds and overtake other probiotic colonies if they are allowed to expand in the body unchecked by probiotic colonies.

This does not seem to be the case during childhood, however. By exposure to soil-based organisms, the young, fresh immune system learns to mount an immune (and probiotic) response that someday may prevent a fatal infection. An adult, on the other hand, may not have the strong immune system the child body once had. As a result, if an adult ingests too many of these organisms, there is the possibility of a significant overgrowth of aggressive and pathogenic bacteria.

This is all a matter of relativity as well. In our antiseptic modern western society, many of our bodies have had little ability to combat and work symbiotically with some of these soil-based organisms. On the other hand, a person who has worked outside in the fields for most of his or her life will likely have a balanced collection of various populations of probiotics and soil-based residents. For these people, a soil-based organism supplement could be an immune-booster. This is the reason that children who are allowed to play outside will have stronger immune systems throughout their lives. If we extend this logic to adults, it is likely that our immune systems will be stronger and more versatile with more time spent outside, gardening for example.

Soil-based organisms also provide a variety of benefits to plants. They are important benefactors for healthy gardens. In the soil, these tiny microbes support plant growth by assisting in the production of a number of nutrients. They also help plants produce phospholipids, which assist and stimulate further plant growth. SBO colonies grow exponentially around roots. Carefully washing fresh plants and roots will dramatically reduce our exposure to these SBOs. At the same time, however, a small amount of exposure to minimal populations during adulthood may be a positive thing, as our immune systems continue to mark and memorize the various organisms that threaten our systems. In addition, a few might end up being transient probiotics. You never know.

A minimal amount of SBO populations, under control, may also help eliminate accumulated putrefaction in intestinal mucosa. *B. subtilis*, for example, was used for centuries by Arabs for dysentery. It was later isolated by the Germans and used for dysentery among the German army during World War II. *B. subtilis* has been the subject of several of clinical trials showing some positive therapeutic responses in some cases.

SBOs have also been observed breaking down hydrocarbons and other molecules, allowing better absorption of difficult-to-digest foods. SBOs can aggressively attack, engulf and ingest other pathogens such as *Candida albicans, Candida parapsilosis, Penicillium frequens, Penicillium notatum, Mucor racemosus, Aspergillus niger* and others. Some SBO strains may work symbiotically with other probiotics. SBOs can also stimulate alpha interferon production. They stimulate "non-addressed" B-lymphocytes, increasing immune response reserves. SBOs also manufacture lactoferrin—iron-binding protein. People who lack lactoferrin may absorb too much iron, which can accumulate around the body, becoming a toxic burden.

Certain SBO strains, such as *Bacillus coagulans* and *B. subtilis,* may be cooperative probiotics at controlled populations, but endospore-forming SBOs in general should be considered more aggressive than probiotic lactobacilli and bifidobacteria species. Minimal colonies—regulated by lactobacilli and bifidobacteria—of these stronger soil-based organisms can help keep our immune systems sharp and responsive. In addition, these stronger soil-based probiotics such as *B. coagulans* and *B. subtilis* can be extremely beneficial during acute infections.

Supplementing Probiotics

One of the misnomers in the probiotic discussion is that probiotic supplementation will result in replacement of resident strains or form permanent colonies. The research, however, has not shown this. The research has so far shown that almost any strain added, either from the diet or through supplementation after the childhood years, will pass through the body within a few days to a couple of weeks.

This does not mean that supplementation has no benefit, as we have seen from the research. Supplemented probiotics change the landscape by reducing pathogenic bacteria and creating a lactic acid fermenting environment that can stimulate growth among our resident strains.

Remember that large genetic differences can exist between different strains of the same probiotic species. Some strains may not colonize well in some people and colonize prolifically in others. This can relate to our existing probiotic colonies, our dietary choices, our stress levels and other environmental issues. For this reason, it is important to experiment with different species, strains and supplement manufacturers to find those that work best for us. As we complete one supplement, we can consider moving to another blend of species and strains. If we find particular success with one brand or formula, we can stick with that too, assuming we are also eating a variety of probiotic foods along with our supplementation. There are some very good quality probiotic supplements available now, and many have a unique assortment of species, strains and culturing methods.

Supplemental probiotic species and strains have typically undergone significant research and testing for safety before they are packaged as supplements. Human-friendly strains are standardized, identified and cataloged within the *American Type Culture Collection* (ATTC) in Manassas, Virginia; or the *Collection*

Nationale de Cultures de Microorganismes at the Institut Pasteur in France. The majority of probiotic supplements sold in the U.S. are (or should be) listed in the ATTC.

It should also be clarified that commercial strains do not always mimic those results found from researched strains. Researchers often uniquely culture a particular strain for the research. The particular culture technique may not equate to those techniques being used for commercial production. Other researchers may use commercial strains, but their handling within the study may not equate to how the commercial strain is handled by the manufacturers, distributors, stores and consumers of those strains.

Finally, as we'll discuss here, some commercial probiotics may be produced, packaged and/or handled in such a way that can cause reductions of viable organisms—through either die-offs or species competition within the formulation.

Supplement Manufacturing Methods

Just as there are a variety of different probiotic species and strains, there are also a number of different methods for producing (culturing) probiotics. Most manufacturers produce probiotics in huge vats or tanks. The vats are mixed with a particular type of medium and starter bacteria. The bacteria are fed for weeks, months or even years (one manufacturer has a three-year process) before they are harvested. Upon harvest, many manufacturers centrifuge the probiotics to strain out the culture. Not all manufacturers centrifuge, however. Some package the substrate medium with their supplement. Still others will use a filtering method. Regardless of the filtering method, most producers then freeze-dry the probiotics into a powder form.

After freeze-drying, the probiotics are typically blended together and packaged, either into capsules, tablets, or shells. Some are mixed with oils, while others are left in powders or mixed into liquids.

Freeze-drying puts microflora into suspended animation. Freeze-dried probiotics are awakened by heat and moisture, however. Once they wake up, they need food and a hospitable environment within which to colonize. If they do not have these available, they will die quickly. For this reason, it is important to keep freeze-dried probiotics enclosed in a dry container or encasing, and preferably in a cool, refrigerated location.

Probiotic manufacturers use a number of delivery vehicles for supplemental probiotics. These come in the form of powders, liquids, capsules, caplets, gums, lozenges and others. Each package has an impact upon probiotic viability and the ability of the supplement to deliver a final 'payload' of colony forming units into the intestines, where the probiotics can thrive and expand.

The first element in probiotic viability is the culturing technique of the manufacturer. Probiotic culturing today is highly advanced. Probiotic manufacturers have developed culture medium advanced formulations and temperature maintanence. These are guarded and technical processes bench-tested in laboratories many years before making it into a production facility. Many producers have patents on their methods, and most keep their methods highly confidential. Viability testing in-house and by third parties create confidence that most ISO-compliant and FDA-inspected producers supply viable freeze-dried probiotics.

Any number of things can go wrong after this. Powders can be left unrefrigerated, and come into contact with moisture. Formulations can mix strains that are not compatible. Encapsulation packaging facilities may be too humid or warm during encapsulation. Finished product in bottles may be left in the sun on a shipping dock, or put on a sunny, heated shelf in the store.

Once probiotics are brought home, they now face new challenges. These can include being left out of the refrigerator. The bottle may be left open, allowing moisture from the air and/or heat to get to the freeze-dried powder. Perhaps a little spray from the faucet gets into the bottle somehow.

Then we come to delivery into the intestines. Here is where it gets really tricky. The probiotic supplement must be in a form that has not only survived all the above threats: It must now somehow deliver the probiotic colony forming units through our stomach's acidity and slip into the intestines to begin colonization. Here the supplement form becomes critical.

Probiotic Supplement Options

Capsules (intestinal): Probiotics come in vegetable, gelatin or enteric-coated capsules. Vegetable capsules contain less moisture than gelatin or enteric-coated capsules. Even a little moisture in the capsule can increase the possibility of waking up the probiotics while in the bottle. Enteric coating can minimally protect the probiotics within the stomach, assuming they have survived in the bottle. Some manufactures use oils to help protect the probiotics in the stomach. In all cases, encapsulated freeze-dried probiotics should be refrigerated (no matter what the label says) at all times during shipping, at the store, and at home. Dark containers are also better protect the probiotics from light.

Powders (intestinal, vaginal, oral): Powders of freeze-dried probiotics are subject to deterioration due to increased exposure to the elements. Powders should be refrigerated in dark containers and sealed tightly to be kept viable. They should also be consumed with liquids or food, preferably dairy or fermented dairy. If used as to insert into the vagina, a douch mixture with water and a little yogurt is preferrable.

Caplets/Tablets (intestinal): The author is aware of one manufacturer producing a caplet with a patented coating shown by lab studies to provide viability through to the intestines without refrigeration. Other tableting systems may also provide protection. If not, those tablets would likely be in the same category as encapsulated products, in terms of requiring refrigeration.

Shells or Beads (intestinal): These can provide longer shelf viability without refrigeration and better survive the stomach.

One drawback is that these can come with less CFU quantity, increasing the cost of a therapeutic dose. Another drawback may be that the intestines must dissolve this thick shell. An easy test is to examine the stool to be sure that the beads or shells aren't coming out the other end whole.

Lozenges, gum and chewable tablets (mouth, nose, throat): These are new and exciting ways to supplement with probiotics. A correctly formulated chewable or lozenge can inoculate the mouth, nose and throat with beneficial bacteria to compete with and fight off pathogenic bacteria as they enter or reside in our nose, throat, mouth and even lungs. This is an excellent way to protect against new infections and prevent sore throats when we are traveling or working in enclosed spaces. The bacteria in a lozenge or chewable ease out as we are sucking or chewing, leaving probiotics dispersed throughout our gums and throat. As we breathe in pathogenic bacteria, these supplemented probiotic bacteria can immediately defend against invasion and potential infection. As indicated in the research covered earlier, oral probiotics can also reduce gum disease such as gingivitis, and reduce dental caries. Manufacturing methods for lozenges and chewables may provide more stability outside of refrigeration. Keeping them sealed, airtight and cool is still a good idea.

Liquid Supplements (intestinal): There are several probiotic supplements in small liquid form. One brand has a long tradition and a hardy, well-researched strain. A liquid probiotic should be in a light-sealed, refrigerated container. It should also contain some dairy or other probiotic-friendly culture, giving the probiotics some food while they are waiting for delivery. One drawback seen by the author is the presence of sugar in some of these products. As we've discussed, simple sugars readily feed pathogenic microorganisms in the gut, such as *Candida spp.*

Probiotic Foods (intestinal and vaginal): There are numerous probiotic foods, including yogurt, kefir, buttermilk and many others. We will discuss in more detail in the next chapter.

Probiotic hydrotherapy inserts (colon): This method of supplementation is probably the best way to implant live colonies of probiotics into the colon. Colon hydrotherapy (or colonic) is one of the healthiest things we can do for preventative and therapeutic health. Colon hydrotherapy is performed by a certified colon hydrotherapist who uses specialized (and sanitary) equipment to flush out the colon and to some degree, the lower intestines. This flushing takes about 30 minutes. Once the process is complete, the hydrotherapist can "insert" a blend of probiotics into the tube and "pump" the probiotics directly into our colon. Colon hydrotherapy is a wonderful treatment recommended for most anyone, especially those with disorders related to autoimmunity, allergies and food sensitivities. Those with sensitive or irritable bowels should consult with their health professional before submitting to a colonic. The one drawback with this method is making an appointment at our local hydrotherapy clinic. The treatments are relatively inexpensive, however. Two to three colonics a year is often recommended for ultimate colon health.

Dosage Considerations

A good dosage for intestinal probiotics for prevention and maintenance can be ten to fifteen billion CFU ("colony forming units") per day, depending upon the packaging and species mix. Total intake during an illness or therapeutic period, however, is often double or triple that dosage. Supplemental oral probiotic dosages can be far less (100 million to 2 billion), especially when the formula contains the hardy *L. reuteri* species.

Travelers can take probiotics before, after and while traveling to avoid infection from strange microbes in foreign food and water. Traveling dosages can be closer to therapeutic doses: 20-30 billion CFU. Oral probiotics are also a good idea for traveling.

Soil-based organisms such as *Bacillus coagulans*, (sometimes incorrectly labeled *Lactobacillus sporogenes*) or *B. subtilis* are often more hardy, and colonize more aggressively in the gut. These spore-forming organisms will also resist stomach acid more than most protein-membrane probiotics. They will, as a result, require smaller doses—such as 500 million to one billion CFU to achieve a therapeutic dose. SBOs like *B. coagulans* may also colonize within the body for a longer duration than a typical, non-spore probiotic species might.

People who must take antibiotics for life-threatening reasons can alternate doses of probiotics between their antibiotic dosing. The probiotic dose can be at least two hours before or after the antibiotic dose. *B. infantis* can be a good supplement of choice for babies. Consult with your prescribing doctor before dosing.

Remember that these dosages depend upon delivery to the intestines. Therefore, a product that passes into the stomach with little protection would likely not deliver well. Such a supplement would likely require higher dosage to achieve the desired effects.

Adhesion and Permanence

Throughout much of five decades of research on probiotics, it has been assumed that those strains that were isolated from human guts and showed advanced adhesion to the intestinal wall become permanent inhabitants of the digestive tract when supplemented.

For example, a study published in 1987 (Conway *et al.*) showed that two strains of *L. acidophilus* and *L. bulgaricus* adhered to the intestinal wall better than other strains of probiotics. This notion of adherence has contributed to the perception that the supplementation of certain strains would render permant populations. This was interpreted by many to mean that supplemented probiotics could replace lost probiotic populations.

However, research that has followed over the years has repeatedly shown that supplemented probiotics rarely if ever become permanent residents. *Never* is a huge leap. The situation would better be described as *no study has proven* that supplemented probiotics become permanent residents. Exceptions may be infants and the elderly. An infant given supplemented probiotics may well harbor some strains as residents, although no studies have confirmed this. In one study, researchers from the National University of Singapore (Mah *et al.* 2007) gave 37 infants *L. rhaminosus* and *B. longum*—both originally derived from humans—for the first six months of life. Once the probiotic supplements were discontinued—even though they were given so early in their lives—the supplemented strains disappeared from their feces. On the other hand, in another study (Szymański *et al.* 2006), a strain of *L. rhamnosus* was found to have "colonized the G.I. tract more persistently," in children with diarrhea.

Most of the research on adults is consistent with this as well. Most has confirmed that supplemented probiotics—even if they were originally isolated from human intestines—will colonize for a week or two within the intestines, and then depart the digestive tract altogether.

How do we know this? Researchers have repeatedly given probiotics while testing stool samples. As they monitor the strains given and excreted, they find that during supplementation, the strains are still colonizing and being excreted. Once the supplementation stops, the strains will continue being excreted for only another 10-12 days. Following this period, there will be little or no sign of the strain whatsoever, indicating that the strain is likely completely removed.

At the same time, research has indicated that the probiotic colonies that propagate our digestive tracts in our first 18 months are the ones that stay with us throughout our lives. These will grow within our digestive tracts and also incubate within our appendix and possibly other regions of the lymphatic system such as the tonsils. They also harbor deep within the mucoid plaque within our digestive tract. Should we knock out thriving colonies with antibiotics, chemicals, or toxins, these incubated strains will be able to colonize and expand as soon as the right environment is re-established.

This means that resident strains of probiotics are likely those that have cultured over generations within our families. They are thus a genetic match for our bodies. The probiotic strains that we receive from our mothers are likely the same strains that we will pass on to our children. Just as our parents' cellular genetics are passed on via the sperm and ovum, our resident probiotics are passed down from mother to child. This means two things: One, our probiotics recognize our cellular genetics as their permanent host environment. Second, our cells and immune system recognizes those strains of probiotics as being residents. This intelligent co-recognition (or cognition) is not so special. After all, our immune system stores and recognizes the identities and characteristics of trillions of different microorganisms—remembering how to handle and defend against each and every one of them should they penetrate the body. Just as we can recognize millions of different faces—our immune system recognizes our probiotics, and our probiotics recognize our immune system.

This commingling and interactive cooperation between our immune system and our probiotics is precisely why our probiotic populations—and those supportive supplemental species— are so critically important to our body's health.

What supplemented probiotics do is set up the environment that stimulates our own strains to begin to re-colonize. The supplemented strains produce lactic acid and nucleic acids and other nutrients that encourage our resident probiotics.

What this all means is that we each have probiotic strains that are unique to us, and to some degree, are shared amongst our families. While we do inherit certain strains, the distinct combination and characteristics, together with subsequent genetic modification among those strains are unique. Just as no DNA is exactly the same from person to person, no collection of probiotic colonies is the same from person to person. In other words, we each have our own special family of probiotic species and strains: Every host and family of probiotics is unique.

Supplementing Probiotics Correctly: Q&A

Let's review and get more specific on the issues surrounding supplementing with probiotics, this time in a question-and-answer format. Excuse any redundancy with previous text, as we attempt to clarify some of these complex topics:

Why, if our body maintains its own resident strains, do we need to take supplemental probiotics?

Cultured and fermented foods have been used for medicinal purposes for several thousand years. Traditional probiotic foods include sauerkraut, pickles, kefir, miso, tempeh, yogurt, kim chi, cheese and kombucha tea. While some of these foods were cultured for taste or preservation, many were found to have substantial benefits for digestive illness. A century ago, Nobel laureate Ilya Mechnikov proposed many of these benefits were derived from supplementing with tiny *Lactobacillus* bacteria that would ferment within a number of probiotic foods.

During the next 100 years, researchers have discovered numerous benefits of probiotic supplementation. Intestinal infections from *Salmonella*, *E. coli*, *Listeria* and other infections have been treated successfully with probiotics. Over the past few decades, research has determined that probiotics produce positive outcomes for a variety of ailments, including ulcers, Crohn's disease, irritable bowel syndrome, candida, constipation, colon cancer, hepatitis and others, as we have discussed.

Probiotics help break down food, attack invading bacteria, and stabilize intestinal walls. Probiotics produce a number of natural antibiotics designed to reduce the populations of invasive yeasts and pathogenic bacteria. They also stimulate the body's own immune system to increase T-cell and B-cell activity.

Most friendly bacteria also produce lactic acid. Lactic acid helps acidify the intestines and prevent harmful bacteria overgrowth. Harmful bacteria manufacture substances that increase the risk of disease by raising the body's toxicity level and even infect the body's joints and organs.

Bifidobacteria make up the large majority of the human body's resident strains. While lactobacilli are considered hardy, aggressive and combative toward invaders, they only comprise about 1% of the body's total probiotic populations.

Once developed, supplemental or food probiotic consumption does not add to our permanent resident populations. Should they make it past our stomach acid, most supplemental or food probiotics pass through our intestinal tracts within about 10-14 days of consumption, assuming supplementation ceases.

This does not mean we only need to take probiotics for two weeks. In fact, therapeutic effects from probiotics typically take longer than eight weeks to accomplish.

Can Probiotic supplements survive production, shipping and handling?

To obtain the most therapeutic results, probiotics must be kept "viable" until they get into the dark and moist environment of our intestines. Most commercial probiotics are cultured in large tanks. Following fermentation, the probiotics are often centrifuged, freeze dried and blended with stabilizers to put them into a state of suspended animation. Any kind of moisture will awaken them from this suspended state. Once awake, they need food and a hospitable environment in order to survive. Without being surrounded by food, they will die. Even if kept in freeze-dried state, probiotics without protection will die if not properly sheltered from moisture and heat.

The process of handling, shipping, packaging and sitting on the shelf can deprive probiotic supplements and probiotic foods of the ability to render health benefits. This is because there are many variables introduced into the packaged probiotics' chain of custody. These possibilities include:

Light: Sunlight or bright light can both wake up and kill probiotics. If they wake up in an environment that does not have enough food, such as in a capsule, the probiotic bacteria will die. Even if the capsule has prebiotics added, this amount will typically not be enough to sustain the probiotics for long.

Heat: Intense heat or immediate temperature change can kill probiotic CFUs. It can also wake up freeze-dried probiotic colonies. In a capsule, this also means sure death from starvation.

Oxygen: Once awake, some probiotics will require oxygen and some will not survive in an oxygen environment. Therefore, if the probiotics awaken from their freeze-dried state, some will die of oxygen exposure and some will die of oxygen debt. Many supplement bottles are nitrogen-filled for this reason.

Vibration: Probiotics are accustomed to the rhythmic motions of intestinal peristalsis. When grown in tanks, they are often stirred to keep some motion going. In a freeze-dried state, this should not be a factor. However, fresh or liquid versions of probiotics may be disrupted by unnatural jostling and handling. Within a fermenting environment such as yogurt or kefir, this should not be a problem, unless there are dramatic temperature changes in addition to drastic motion changes. Nonetheless, shaking of a probiotic drink should be done gently.

Practically any encapsulated probiotic will require refrigeration for CFU viability, even if the label says otherwise. There are only a few probiotic supplement forms on the market today that do not require refrigeration (that the author is aware of). These are the enclosed shells and the tablets containing a patented intestinal delivery system. This should be evident from the label.

Not surprisingly, a number of studies and consumer reports have confirmed that many probiotic supplements contain far less viable organisms than listed on their labels. Refrigerated probiotic products faired far better in these tests than did non-refrigerated products. Still, many refrigerated products also showed levels far lower than quantities listed on their labels.

What are the best probiotic brands to buy?

Most probiotic brands are contract-manufactured. This means that the owners of the brand—often the formulators—are not the producers of the product. They contract the production with another company—usually a company that is specifically skilled in the manufacturing and shipping of probiotics. This does not mean that the probiotic contract-packed products are bad. This can be a good thing in some cases. However, it also means that whoever may have developed the formula and wrote the label may not be significantly experienced in the field of probiotics.

For this reason, we often see probiotic products that are not properly labeled, and we see formulas that have competitive strains or too many strains. We also often find labels that say "Refrigeration Not Needed" when refrigeration is needed. We also find instances when the label instructs the person to take the probiotic on an empty stomach, when the stomach is at its peak of acid production and most likely to destroy many of the viable organisms.

In 1990, Natasha Trenev proposed Good Manufacturing Practices and labeling standards for probiotic manufacturers to the newly formed Probiotic Interest Group of the National Nutritional Foods Association (NNFA). After being approved by a vote of the committee for the Natural Products Quality Assurance Alliance (NPQAA), these standards established guidelines for the manufacture and labeling of probiotics.

Unfortunately, because these standards have been voluntary, they are not always practiced. As a result, many of the brands and labels found on today's shelves fall below these standards. As a result, we find a variety of different types of probiotic labeling, which serves to confuse consumers comparing brands.

As hinted at above, there have been several studies published over the past three decades on probiotic products. In a 1985 study published in the *Journal of Alternative and Complemen-*

tary Medicine, it was found that several brands had far fewer CFU counts than was stated on the label. Probiotic research at the University of Nebraska has tested more than 200 acidophilus products over a 20-year period. Of these, 70-80% had less CFU counts than claimed on the label, and almost 50% had less than 10% of the viable CFU counts claimed on the labels.

In 2005, *Consumer Reports* published a study that rated a number of brands of supplements and yogurts. Once again, it was found that several supplement brands that had CFU counts less than stated on the labels. They also found that several natural yogurts had significantly greater CFU counts than did many of the supplements.

These studies have rendered a significant challenge to probiotic manufacturers. In recent years, some manufacturers have responded by developing increasingly better production and handling methods (as mentioned above) to accomplish a greater number of viable organisms.

Here are a few points about labeling products to consider:

❖ The strain quantities should be in colony forming units (CFU). Many brands will list the probiotics as milligrams, which does not indicate the viable (living) quantities.

❖ Many products state CFU potency at the manufacturing date. This is no guarantee of the product's potency at the time of purchase, however. This does not necessarily mean these products don't have good potency. It just means the potency might be less than what is stated on the label. New regulations coming into play will require that CFU counts be guaranteed through the date of expiration. It will soon become obvious which brands have qualified CFU counts.

❖ Many encapsulated brands claim no refrigeration is necessary for freeze-dried powered probiotics. Most studies and experts agree that a freeze-dried probiotic—in any type of capsule—should be refrigerated to keep its viability. If the product is powdered or in a capsule and it is not refrigerated at the store, it may be a "dud."

❖ There are a few brands that have either specially-coated caplets (a special intestinal delivery mechanism) or a thick shell around them. Manufacturer tests state that these retain viability without refrigeration.

❖ Exceptions to this are a few spore-forming types of "soil-based" bacteria, such as *Bacillus coagulans*—often mislabeled as *L. sporongenes.* These are hardy enough to live for a reasonable amount of time outside of refrigeration without a medium.

❖ Some brands have been formulated and backed up by professionals who are skilled in probiotic formulation. A look at the brand's website will usually reveal how much expertise they have.

Can supplemented probiotics survive stomach acids to get to the intestines?

Probiotics need to get into our intestines to do our digestive systems any good. Should they survive the stresses of production, shipping and handling, and no one in the supply chain left encapsulated product out of the refrigerator; the probiotics will still have to survive the acids of the stomach to give us any credible benefit in the intestines.

This means they need to be in a form that protects them from stomach acids. (This does not apply to oral probiotic lozenges, however. Their intended delivery is made once we pop them into our mouths.)

Sadly, most commercial delivery systems for probiotic supplements and foods do not adequately shield the microorganisms from the destructive forces of stomach acid. Once removed from its culture and centrifuged, the microorganism is left without much protection. Stomach acid, in fact, is designed to repel bacteria.

Powders of course, are exposed immediately to stomach acid. Vegetable and gelatin capsules are designed to immediately dissolve in the presence of heat and moisture. This means they will dissolve in the stomach quite easily. For this reason, enteric-coated capsules have become popular, but these may also be dissolved in a healthy stomach acid environment.

This means that we should also consider how the probiotics are packaged otherwise. Are they encapsulated with a protective medium such as oil or culture? Or perhaps packed into shells or coated caplets? These extra steps create more assurancees of viability through to the intestines.

Should we take probiotics with meals or between meals?

This depends upon the strain and the form of the probiotic supplement. A well-coated or otherwise oil-bound probiotic supplement (not just encapsulated or enteric coated) can be taken between meals to speed its entry into the intestinal tract. But for typical encapsulated freeze-dried versions, it is probably best to have the alkalizing effect of food helping to buffer the stomach acids. Better to take these with or following meals.

L. bulgaricus is particularly better when taken with food, as it is more sensitive to stomach acids than other species.

In other words, some probiotic supplements may be better taken on an empty stomach, but these are limited to those made with a considerable amount of protection: Like the intestinal delivery caplets, the shells, or the oil-packaged formulations. Because these can better survive stomach acids, the probiotics will easily be delivered directly into the intestines.

We should consider, however, that once awakened in the moist environment of our intestines, probiotics need food. Therefore, a probiotic supplement should be taken amongst a diet of prebiotic or cultured probiotic foods. This way, the probiotics will have plenty of good nutrition once they awaken from their dormancy.

What about probiotic foods?

Probiotic food formulations are increasingly showing up in our grocery stores. Many foods now claim to be "probiotic foods." Are they really?

Yogurt and kefir are both tremendous probiotic foods. This is because their live bacteria will "culture" or feed off the milk and continue to live for many months, assuming refrigeration following the 24-48 hour incubation period. Tests have illustrated that a large cup of quality yogurt can contain a several hundred million to several billion viable and living CFUs, while supplemented yogurt can have several billion. As to whether probiotics in yogurt and kefir bacteria survive the stomach acid, this will depend upon our stomach's acidity and the cultured medium. Because they are fermenting within the protective medium of cultured dairy, yogurt and kefir probiotics have a good opportunity to penetrate the intestines, and studies on intestinal disorders that used yogurt have supported this.

What about those brands with one special strain of organism? These may work well, depending upon how hardy the strain is. Some of the newly patented strains have been shown in studies to be hardy and productive. One problem with some yogurts however, may be amount of refined sugar content. Unlike oligosaccharides and fructooligosaccharides—stacked saccharides that probiotics feed from—refined sugars will feed the yeasts and spore-forming competitors of probiotics, which may be counterproductive to our probiotic strategy.

Making homemade cultures or buying plain organic cultured foods are probably the best strategies for probiotic foods. Several natural and organic yogurt brands have a high level of integrity and a greater awareness of probiotic survival. Organic fermented products like yogurt, kefir, kombucha and cheese are typically produced by manufacturers focused upon culturing their foods in a manner that continues the probiotic traditions of our ancestors. We'll discuss probiotic foods in more detail later.

Which strains should I choose?

Over the past century, many probiotic species and strains of those species have been isolated from various mediums. As a result, the American Type Culture Collection in Manassas Virginia and the Collection Nationale de Cultures de Microorganismes at the Institut Pasteur in France are crammed with hundreds of registered probiotic strains, many accompanying clinical research showing benefits to humans.

Some of these strains have been patented by the discoverer. Some have also had their names trademark-registered.

Earlier we laid out the major species—those most used in supplements—and their effects according to human research. Within each species, however, are a variety of subspecies and strains. As we've discussed, research has established that some strains may be hardier and more productive than certain other strains of that same species.

Fifty years ago, Khem Shahani, Ph.D., a professor at the University of Nebraska-Lincoln, led research teams that isolated a variety of probiotic strains from human intestines. Among those were several *Lactobacillus acidophilus* strains that appeared to be hardier than others. The DDS line of strains (DDS is an acronym for Department of Dairy Sciences, later changed to the Department of Food Sciences and Technology) were notable for their high gut implantation rates and longer survival rates in their research. As the research continued, some of these DDS strains showed better implantation rates. Dr. Shahani wrote in his scientific writings that because DDS, "was isolated from a human source, it is exceedingly well accepted by the human body, implanting and multiplying in the intestinal tract more easily than flora from animal strains, such as those used to make yogurt and some other flora supplements."

We should note that much of Dr. Shahani's research occurred a few decades ago, and many other strains of *Lactobacillus acidophilus* have been isolated (some also from the human gut) by researchers since. Some have also been patented and trademark-registered, just as some of the DDS strains have. Many others have been isolated and left in the public domain for any manufacturer to use without paying licensing fees.

Some isolated strains have been identified as "super strains" because of their success in the research. This is likely part science and part marketing. These strains are easily recognized in the human research reviewed earlier, and their effects are evident.

However, generic probiotic strains that have been isolated (some also from humans) over the years may well be as implantable and effective as the patented and/or trademarked strains. The research is simply not organized enough, and there are simply too many strains out there to know concretely how well some isolated strains stack up against all the other possible strains of that species. In fact, it is entirely likely that some of us will receive some strains positively that others do not. There are billions of unique strains of each type of species that inhabit our inner and outer environments. Each will have a slightly different DNA, and slightly different characteristics.

Put it this way: While there is plenty of research showing some strains are more vigorous than others, this author knows of no specific research that confirms that a particular strain is the only strain of that species with the particular effects found among studies of a specific strain. As evidenced by some of the research reviewed in this book, we see different strains of the same species produce the same or similar effects when supplemented. From this fact alone, we can logically surmise that the patented strains are not the only strains that should produce those effects. At the same time, as mentioned above, some strains have certainly been found to be more resilient and productive than certain other strains of the same species. This is the reason for some of these strains being patented and/or trademarked.

For example, University of Nebraska research showed a number of *L. acidophilus* strains—labeled with DDS numbers—

were more resilient than certain other *L. acidophilus* strains. But did he test every possible strain of *L. acidophilus*? Certainly not. At one time, there were about 200 *L. acidophilus* strains known. Today we know there are many more.

Studies with comparisons of effects between large numbers of multiple strains of the same species are few if not non-existent. There is currently little incentive for such a costly and thorough study. Therefore, there is little conclusive evidence a patented strain is better than all other strains of the same species. Comparisons certainly have been done on a small or commercial scale or between a few strains of the same species—which is worth some consideration as we choose between strains. But the author is unaware of any conclusive comparison in the form of a peer-reviewed clinical study of a significantly large number of different strains of the same species—patented or not.

Nearly all probiotics will inhibit intestinal infections to one degree or another. Nearly all will help with irritable bowels and other intestinal issues. However, as we saw from the research we reviewed, some probiotic *species* will produce benefits that other *species* do not produce. This we can be sure of.

Some brands and manufacturers utilize only those strains that have been the subject of clinical research. This is a practical approach, as we can follow that strain back to the research. We can have more confidence that the strain produces the effects we are looking for. On the other hand, some manufacturers do not utilize those specific strains, because they are patented and thus require licensing fees to be paid to the company that holds the patent. This cost is surely passed on to the consumer.

This means that a generic strain of the same species may cost significantly less to the consumer. Does this mean the product will not accomplish the same results as those found in the research on different strains of that species? Some experts feel the patented strains are no better than the generic species. Others feel the patented strains are worth the extra money because they have been proven effective in the study. Regardless of the position, the situation cannot be compared to generic drugs—which are often identical in molecular formula to the branded drug.

The other wild card to consider is that the fermentation medium used for the culturing of the probiotics used in the clinical research may vastly differ from the medium used by the commercial manufacturer—even if the manufacturer is using the same strain as the research. In reality, the medium of fermentation is just as critical as the strain. In other words, a bacteria fermented in a milk medium could differ in activity from a bacteria fermented in a soymilk medium or a broth medium.

Even within milk mediums, we find there are a variety of methods and types of milk being used, from skim milk to whole fat milk and many shades between. Then there is organic milk, pasteurized milk and more. Some researchers may have fermented their probiotic strains in a unique combination of milk and FOS, for example. These unique methods will yield bacteria that may respond quite differently from those of the same strain cultured in a large manufacturing facility.

Speaking of FOS, some probiotic supplements also contain prebiotics, providing immediate food for the bacteria. This may slightly improve survival and colonization, or change the virility of the bacteria in general, but this is fairly unlikely for a freeze-dried product.

There is also reason to believe that a likely mechanism for the effects produced by many probiotics is the removal of pathogenic bacteria and the preparation of the intestinal 'turf' for our own resident strains to re-colonize and re-establish their former glory as our immune system companions. Because probiotic supplementation studies have illustrated boosts in strains that were not supplemented, it is logical to assume that those 'other' strains are actually our resident families that have been able to rebuild their previous territorial positions. We'll discuss this possibility a little more later.

All of this might be quite dizzying to the consumer. The best thing to do is conduct some research on the manufacturer, the product label, the branding company, and the formulation expertise behind the product. This will usually yield good decisions regarding the brand to use.

Even then, it can make sense to switch from one probiotic brand to another every so often. Another brand or manufacturer's culturing methods may result in more probiotic viability. Another brand may have better handling methods. If we do decide to switch, however, it is best to finish the entire bottle, unless we are finding that the product is not effective at all. In that case, we should consider returning the product to the store or seller.

The reason to finish the bottle is twofold. First, probiotics do not have long shelf lives, so it is best to save any for a later date. Secondly, it is best to provide enough CFU strength over a period of time for those strains to colonize and make a territorial dent in their new environment and among the immune system.

In terms of number of strains in a supplement, we need to remember that different species of bacteria will compete. This means that too many species, or the wrong species combinations, could result in only one or two "conquering" strains being left in the supplement at the time of use. This was evidenced in some laboratory studies in the 1980s. Too many organism strains can also compete in the gut, creating uncertain outcomes: Best to take no more than four or five different probiotic strains at a time, including at least one *Lactobacillus* and one *Bifidobacterium* strain. Careful selection of strains, supplement packaging and food brands can make the difference between significantly boosting our immune system and wasting our money.

We should note also that there are a few species that are more vigorous than others. This is the case with the *L. casei* strain. Manufacturer research on combination probiotic products has determined that a combination formula with *L. casei* can result in the *L. casei* overtaking the other strains in the product. In some cases, this may not be a bad thing, however. As we saw in the research, the *L. casei* strain can be highly productive.

This may be a problem if we are trying to supplement both our lactobacilli and bifidobacteria species, however. *L. casei* may overtake the bifidobacteria in the supplement, for example. Therefore, it is probably best to take *L. casei* by itself if we want to specifically obtain the effects of *L. casei*.

Another vigorous bacteria species is *Enterococcus faecium*. This species is obviously classified as enterococci, and some of the strains in this class are pathogenic. Still other strains in this species have been isolated and found to be probiotic, and these we have discussed. Combinations that contain *E. faecium* should be approached cautiously, however. The product may end up being mostly *E. faecium* in content.

It is probably best to utilize those species whose different strains have undergone the most research. This will give us some assurance that these species are safer and more productive in the human environment.

The most researched species include ones listed in the previous chapter. Of colon-happy bifidobacteria, these include *Bifidobacterium bifidum*, *B. infantis*, *B. longum*, *B. lactis* and *B. breve*. For the intestines, we see *Lactobacillus acidophilus*, *L. salivarius*, *L. casei*, *L. rhamnosus*, *L. reuteri*, *L. plantarum*, *L. bulgaricus* and *L. brevis* have the most research. Others include *Streptococcus thermophilus* and *Enterococcus faecium*. Researched probiotic yeasts include *Saccharomyces boulardii* and *Saccharomyces cerevisiae*.

For the mouth, *Lactobacillus acidophilus*, *L. salivarius*, *L. reuteri*, and *L. plantarum* have undergone the most research.

Among the soil-based spore-formers, *Bacillus coagulans* and *Bacillus subtilis* have undergone the most clinical human research. These have both been shown to be safe, and have shown to be especially functional in chronically diseased states. Other soil-based organisms or SBOs (also sometimes called HSOs) may not be as healthy. They may, in fact, become pathogenic bacteria if they are allowed to overgrow other populations.

It is also for this reason that probiotic supplements and foods combined with SBOs will often show greater plate counts—and seemingly more viable organisms than other probiotic supplements or foods. In many of these cases, the rigorous spore-forming bacteria may have taken over the probiotic content of the supplement or food. What remains could be similar to a supplement with only the SBO organisms. While this population may be beneficial to certain people and certain conditions, the probiotic food or supplement may not contain the well-rounded group of probiotics indicated on the label.

How much and for how long?

Again, dosages for probiotics depend on the strain, combination and condition. Clinical evidence has illustrated that the dosage needs to be large enough to create a suitable environment for the implantation of probiotic colonies. This also depends upon the product. For most encapsulated, refrigerated products, most experts recommend between 15-40 billion CFU per day as a therapeutic dose for a couple of months, and 5-15 billion per day as a follow-up/maintenance dose. This maintenance dose should be ongoing—at least for a year or two. After that time, the dosage can be variable—a week or two straight, then a week or two off. Some of the clinical studies utilized dosages of more than 40 billion CFU per day to achieve their therapeutic results.

This also assumes a small mix of 3-4 probiotics that are compatible. For coated caplets or shells, dosages can halve these, as more of these should reach the intestines.

Many commercial product labels recommend far less dosages. These can range from a 3-5 billion CFU for some, and even from 750 million to 1.5 billion CFU per day for others. These might be particularly hardy strains, or spore-forming strains such as *B. subtilis/L. sporongenes*, or formulations that include the lactic acid fermentation medium into the product. For the common strains and typical packaging types—such as lactobacilli and bifidobacteria in capsules—these dosage levels would be likely be less than therapeutic.

How do I know the probiotics are effective?

After a few days of supplementation, we should see a change in our feces. We should find that our stool becomes more firm and less loose. Our stool should take on defined aerodynamic missile shapes with smooth contours and little water. Our bowel movements should also become easier. While some might contend that healthy stool should float, this depends greatly upon the fiber, fat and the rest of the content of our diet.

The effects upon our stool should come within a week or two after dosing—or longer for those with chronic intestinal problems. Other beneficial effects can take several months of consistent dosing to observe. As we read in the research reviewed earlier, most of the successful studies used treatment periods of eight weeks or more. Many studies treated their subjects for several months. Some even treated for a year or two. These longer studies have often shown greater levels of success.

The other way to tell that probiotics are effective is that we should have less flatulence, less bloating, and less indigestion. After a few weeks, we might also see improvements in our skin complexion, our moods, and our immune systems. These effects may be so subtle that we may not realize what caused them. Results may also be slow, and require perserverance to achieve.

Good judgment is part of deciding how to dose probiotics. Dosages depend on the strain, formula, packaging, and condition. First, the dosages need to be large enough to properly acidify the intestines. Second, they must be large enough to repel invading organisms. Third, they must be sufficient enough for sizeable colonies to attach to our intestinal walls and begin to work their magic on our immune system.

Should children supplement with probiotics?

This is an important question. As we saw in the research on infants, probiotic supplementation can greatly stimulate the immune system, create better nutrition, fight off infection and stimulate growth among children. However, there can be a few downsides.

Supplemental probiotics may be competitive to the initial strains that mother gives the child. A healthy mother will be giving the child probiotics during vaginal delivery and breast-feeding. These two functions accompany more than just the delivery of probiotics. Baby also receives a variety of nutrients and immunoglobulins from the vagina birth and breast-feeding. Baby needs to have these successfully implant into the digestive tract and immune system. Too many vigorous supplemented probiotics too early may interfere in this process.

For example, *B. subtilus* and *L. bulgaricus* present a particular form of lactic acid—with the D+ bonding format—that can inhibit the growth of *B. infantis* bacteria. *B. infantis* is the central *Bifidobacterium* that implants into the colon to set up the mechanisms of cholesterol release and the bile salt exchange with the liver. *B. infantis* sets up shop and creates a particular type of lactic acid environment—with the L+ bonding format. Therefore, one should be careful in choosing the strains supplemented to infants.

Should the infant be birthed through a ceasarian and/or not be breast-fed, then supplementing with *B. infantis* initially, and then adding *L. acidophilus* and *B. bifidus* after a few weeks or months may be appropriate. After a few months, other strains may be cautiously added in small doses. In all cases, the parent should consult with a health professional knowledgeable in probiotic supplementation to children, preferably one with a clinical understanding of the child's needs.

Living With Our Probiotics

After researchers at University of Rome's School of Medicine (Pagnini *et al.* 2008) studied the relationship between probiotics and the development of colon cancer, they described probiotic activity as "oncologic surveillance." This was because the researchers realized that probiotics somehow became aware of a developing tumor, and then stimulated the process of cytotoxic action—killing the tumor cells.

What this means is that our probiotics are looking out for our bodies. They are watching our cells and tissue systems. When they perceive some threat to their home, they will work to remove it, while signaling the immune system for support.

We might compare this activity to how we might care for the environment around our house. We will cultivate our soil, plant nice trees, and pull weeds, all in an effort to create a pleasing, comfortable environment. When a mole or a deer gets into the yard, we will shoo them away for fear that they might chew up our plants or otherwise ruin the nice surroundings we have been cultivating.

The research indicates that probiotics are no different. Our resident strains cultivate a good, healthy environment within their life-long host. Supplemented probiotics will also set up housekeeping, even though they are transients. We might compare supplemented probiotics to going on vacation. Even though we will only be staying in our hotel room for a week, we will still keep it at a comfortable temperature, keep out the flies and mosquitoes, and keep it neat and clean so that while we are staying there, our quarters are comfortable for us and our colony—er, family.

Now if someone or something were to threaten our home or even our hotel room, we will immediately react. We would call the police, or even prepare our own defense measures.

These kinds of tendencies are universal among all living organisms. We see birds creating their nests, and then standing guard and chirping others away from their territory. We see dogs taking care of their masters and barking at any possible threats. We see bears burrowing into their sleeping spaces and clearing them out, and covering them for protection against invaders. Even plants and trees are territorial. Most trees, for example, will produce particular biochemicals in their saps and leaves that repel the growth of insects, burrowing animals, and even other plants. This is because every living being has an innate desire to survive comfortably.

Probiotics are no different.

Conscious and territorial creatures living within our bodies might seem odd, but we also see other symbiotic behavior between species throughout nature. Species that take care of each other are simply working for their own ongoing survival.

Because probiotics take such good care of us, it only makes sense for us to take care of their survival as well. This means we need to look carefully at our lifestyles and our eating behavior and address whether we are maintaining a sustainable environment for our families of probiotics. We need to look at whether we are providing our probiotics a habitat that helps them flourish. We know from the research that if their colonies flourish, our bodies will be healthier and our immune systems will be stronger. So what can we do to promote strong colonization among our probiotic friends?

The Probiotic Friendly Diet

Our health depends not just upon different populations of probiotics surviving within our bodies: They must thrive and colonize to the greatest extent. This allows their colonies to be strong enough to counter any invading pathogen. A weak probiotic colony is not much better than no colony, because it will be easily conquered in an invasion.

Even if some of these thriving colonies are transient, they will still be territorial, as the research has indicated. They will also be producing nutrients, helping us digest our foods and keeping pathogenic bacteria populations at bay. As supplemented or transient strains grow, they also prepare our system for the regrowth of our resident strains.

For example, it appears evident that diet and healthy probiotic colonies are directly related to the avoidance of colon cancer and other intestinal disease. In 1980, Dr. Barry Goldin and fellow researchers reported a series of studies that connected certain diets with a group of enzymes found to be involved in the incidence of cancer. These enzymes were beta-glucuronidase, nitroreductase, azoreductase, and steroid 7-alpha-dehydroxylase.

Incidentally, studies with vegetarians have found lower levels of these enzymes, while meat-eaters have greater levels. Apparently, these cancer-related enzymes seem to have their origin from the presence of pathogenic bacteria in the intestines. It has become increasingly evident that these carcinogenic and pathogenic enzymes are endotoxins from pathogenic bacteria.

This led Dr. Goldin and associates to study the difference between these enzyme levels in omnivores and vegetarians. The researchers removed meat from the diets of a group of omnivores for 30 days. A reduction of steroid 7-alpha-dehydroxylase was found. With the addition of *L. acidophilus* supplementation, however, this group also showed a significant reduction in beta-glucuronidase and nitroreductase.

Furthermore, other studies, some of which we reviewed earlier, have confirmed that various probiotic bacteria reduce levels of beta-glucuronidase. Beta-glucuronidase is one of the enzymes most associated with colon cancer in cancer research. In Dr. Golden's research, thirty days after the withdrawal of the *L. acidophilus* supplementation, the enzymes returned to previous (unhealthy) levels.

Two years later, Dr. Goldin and associates (Goldin *et al.* 1982) studied 10 vegetarian and 10 omnivore women. He found that the vegetarian women produced significantly lower levels of beta-glucuronidase than the omnivorous women—a result that was unrelated to the supplementation of probiotics or any other treatments.

The association between colon cancer and red meat has been shown conclusively in a variety of studies over the years. In an American Cancer Society cohort study (Chao *et al.* 2005) of 148,610 adults between the ages of 50 and 74 living in 21 states, higher intakes of red and processed meats were associated with higher levels of rectal and colon cancer after other cancer variables were eliminated.

Other studies have confirmed the depletion of carcinogenic enzymes produced by pathogenic bacteria in vegetarian diets. Researchers from Finland's University of Kuopio (Ling and Hanninen 1992) tested 18 volunteers who were randomly divided into either a control group (conventional animal products diet) or an extreme vegan diet for one month, followed by the return to the original omnivore diet. After only one week on the vegan diet, the researchers found that fecal urease levels decreased by 66%, cholylglycine hydrolase levels decreased by 55%, beta-glucuronidase levels decreased by 33% and beta-glucosidase levels decreased by 40% in the vegan group, and continued through the month of consuming the vegan diet. Serum levels of phenol and p-cresol—also endotoxins of pathogenic bacteria—also significantly decreased in the vegan group. Within two weeks of returning to the animal diet, all of the pathogenic fecal enzyme levels returned to the levels before converting to the vegan diet. After one month of returning to the omnivore diet, the serum levels of toxins phenol and p-cresol returned to their previously higher levels prior to the vegan diet. Meanwhile, no changes in any of these enzymes or toxin levels occurred among the conventional (omnivore diet) control group.

A study published two years earlier by Huddinge University researchers (Johansson *et al.* 1990) also confirmed the same results. The conversion of an omnivore diet to a lacto-vegetarian diet significantly reduced levels of beta-glucuronidase, beta-glucosidase, and sulphatase from fecal samples.

Another study illustrating this link between vegetarianism, pathogenic bacterial enzymes and cancer was conducted at Sweden's Huddinge University and the University Hospital (Johansson *et al.* 1998) almost a decade later. Dr. Johansson and associates measured the effect of switching from an omnivore diet to a lacto-vegetarian diet and back to an omnivore diet with respect to mutagenicity: testing the body's fluid biochemistry to determine the tendency for tumor formation. Twenty non-smoking and normal weight volunteers switched to a lacto-vegetarian diet for one year. Urine and feces were examined for mutagenicity (mutagenic bacteria and endotoxins) at the start of the study, at three months, at six months and at twelve months after beginning the vegetarian diet. Following the switch to the lacto-vegetarian diet, all mutagenic parameters significantly decreased among the urine and feces of the subjects. The subjects were then tested once more, three years after converting back to an omnivore diet. The mutagenic biochemistry levels returned.

The clear conclusion we must take away from this research is that probiotics prefer vegetarian diets, and vegetarian diets inhibit the growth of pathogenic bacteria that create a cancer-friendly environment. Since the levels of these enzymes fall significantly following the addition of probiotics, we can correlate that probiotics are involved in removing and controlling the pathogenic bacteria that produce these enzymes. Because beta-glucuronidase levels are higher in an omnivore diet, we can conclude that eating meat discourages the growth of probiotics and encourages the growth of pathogenic bacteria that produce these cancer-friendly enzymes. We can also then conclude that since vegetarians produce lower levels of beta-glucuronidase and other pathogenic, cancer-related enzymes, vegetarian diets also must promote probiotic growth and decrease the risk of colon cancer.

A contributing mechanism of this effect was found in Dr. Goldin's 1982 research, and confirmed by other research on vegetarians since. Vegetarian diets promote faster fecal excretion cycles than do meat diets. In other words, vegetarian meals move through the digestive tract faster, and meat meals move through slower. This means that a meat diet allows for more time for pathogenic bacteria to colonize. In addition, meat diets introduce into the digestive system new populations of pathogenic bacteria. This later point is confirmed by the numerous foodborne outbreaks associated with commercial meat products.

Probiotic Nourishment: Prebiotics

One of the most important factors in establishing a healthy environment for our probiotic colonies is making sure they have the right mix of nutrients available. The nutrients our probiotic families favor are called prebiotics. In other words, some foods are particularly beneficial for *bifidobacteria, lactobacilli* and other probiotic populations. These are the oligosaccharides, fructooligosaccharides, galactooligosaccharides, and transgalactooligosaccharides—also referred to as inulin, FOS, GOS and TOS. Even two or three grams of one of these prebiotics will dramatically increase *bifidobacteria* populations assuming resident colonies. Inulin, FOS, GOS and TOS are also antagonistic to toxic microorganism genera such as *Salmonella, Listeria, Campylobacter, Shigella* and *Vibrio*. These and other pathogenic bacteria tend to thrive from refined sugars as opposed to the complex saccharides of inulin, FOS, GOS and TOS.

Oligosaccharides are short stacks of simple yet mostly indigestible sugars (from the Greek *oligos*, meaning "few"). If the sugar molecule is fructose, the stacked molecule is called a fructooligosaccharide. If the sugar molecule is galactose, the stacked molecule is called a galactooligosaccharide. These molecules are very useful for human cells and probiotics because they can be processed directly for energy as well as be combined with fatty acids to create cell wall structures and cellular communication molecules. These nutrients also provide energy and nourishment to our probiotic colonies.

The oligosaccharides inulin and oligofructose are probably the most recognized prebiotics. Inulin is a naturally occurring carbohydrate used by plants for storage. It has been estimated that more than 36,000 plant species contain inulin in varying degrees (Carpita *et al.* 1989). The roots often contain the greatest amounts of inulin.

Commercial sources of inulin include Jerusalem artichoke, agave cactus and chicory. Chicory, the root of the Belgian endive, is known to contain some of the highest levels of both inulin at 15-20%, and oligofructose at 5-10%. Inulin from agave has been described as highly branched. This gives it a higher solubility and digestibility than inulin derived from Jerusalem artichoke or chicory.

Notable prebiotic FOS-containing foods include beets, leeks, bananas, tree fruits, soybeans, burdock root, asparagus, maple sugar, whole rye and whole wheat among many others. Bananas contain one of the highest levels of FOS. Bananas are thus a favorite food for both humans and probiotics.

GOS and TOS are natural byproducts of milk. They are produced as lactose is enzymatically converted or hydrolyzed within the digestive tract. This process can also be done commercially. Before much of the recent research on GOS was performed, nutritionists simply thought of GOS and TOS as indigestible byproducts of milk.

Another element in plant foods providing prebiotic nutrition for probiotics is the polyphenol group. Polyphenols are groups of biochemicals produced in plants such as lignans, tannins, reservatrol, and flavonoids. There is some uncertainty as to which of these are most helpful to probiotic populations.

Some prebiotics have interesting side effects. For example, there seems to be a relationship between oligofructose inulin and calcium absorption. Inulin has been shown to improve calcium absorption by 20%, and yogurt supplemented with TOS has increased calcium absorption by 16% (van den Heuvel *et al.* 2000)

Galactooligosaccharides have another side effect that is important to note. Dr. Kari Shoaf and fellow researchers at the University of Nebraska (Shoaf *et al.* 2006) found in laboratory tests that galactooligosaccharides reduce the ability of *E. coli* to attach to human cells within tissue cultures. This effect was isolated from GOS' ability to nourish probiotics. This means that GOS provides more than nutrition to our probiotic colonies. This once considered useless indigestible nutrient also helps keep *E. coli* and other pathogenic bacteria from attaching to our cells. A nice package deal indeed.

FOS and GOS have been known to cause digestive disturbance in rare cases. Such a digestive disturbance is likely caused by dysbiosis, however.

Conclusively, a preponderance of scientific literature indicates that probiotics thrive from a diet of plant-based natural foods with plenty of phytonutrients, while overly processed, sugary and meat diets tend to promote pathogenic bacteria and their disease-causing endotoxins.

Probiotic Hydration

Our probiotics need water just as our bodies do. Our intestinal tract requires sufficient water for our gastric cells and intestinal wall cells to function properly. Like our bodies, the body of a probiotic is mostly water. Water thus serves as a critical nutrient for our microflora friends. Probiotics also require a wet environment to maintain their movement, communications and colonization processes. We should also remember that prebiotics are fibrous, and thus require water to move them through the digestive tract.

The question is how much water is necessary? Conventional advice has suggested around six to eight 8-oz glasses per day for an adult. However, in 2004, the National Academy of Sciences released a study indicating that the average woman requires approximately 91 ounces of water per day, while men meet their needs with about 125 ounces per day. This study also indicated that approximately 80% of this comes from drinking water and beverages, and 20% comes from food. Therefore, we can assume a minimum of 73 ounces of fresh water/beverages for the average adult woman and 100 ounces of fresh water/beverages for the average adult man should cover our minimum needs. That is significantly more water than the standard eight glasses per day (64 ounces)—especially for men. It is not surprising that some health professionals have suggested that 50-75% of Americans suffer from chronic dehydration. Fereydoon Batmanghelidj, M.D. (1997), one of the world's most respected researchers on human hydration, suggests 1/2 ounce of water per pound of body weight. For those who exercise (also good for probiotic colonies) an additional 8-16 ounces for each forty-five minutes to an hour of strenuous activity would be suggested. This is best taken before and after exercising, in addition to taking a few sips during the workout. Extremes in temperature and elevation increase our water requirements as well. Additional water is also required during periods of fever or increased sweating.

Hydration experts agree that as soon as we feel thirsty, our bodies are already experiencing dehydration. Becoming consciously thirsty is the point where tissue and probiotic damage is occurring. Our thirst sensation decreases as we age, so it is much easier to become dehydrated in our later years. Water is critical for the smooth running of all of our cells. Tissues likely to suffer first during dehydration include our digestive tract, joints, eyes and liver. Some health experts have estimated as little as a 5%

loss of body water will decrease physical performance by up to 30%. We should also watch our urine to be sure we are getting enough water. Our urine color should range from light yellow to clear. Darker urine indicates dehydration.

Synbiotics

The blending of probiotics with prebiotics is called synbiotics. This is an increasingly relevant strategy for probiotic use. Dehydrated FOS, inulin and combinations thereof have been popularized in a number of successful probiotic supplements and food formulations. To this we can add that most properly fermented dairy products such as yogurt or kefir should already have an ample supply of GOS and/or TOS available to nourish our incoming probiotic friends.

We should understand the importance of having prebiotics available to probiotics during their transit. Most probiotic supplements are freeze-dried prior to encapsulation or shipment. This means that they have been put into incubation—a sort of sleep mode. As soon as they come into contact with a little water or heat, they will wake up. Once they wake up, like any living being after hibernation, they will be hungry.

If the newly awakened bacterium does not have enough prebiotic food available immediately, it will soon die. This is why many probiotics die within the supplement before they even get into our bodies. Often the capsule will contain a little moisture, or some light or heat will heat up the bottle. This awakens the probiotic, who then must find some food or face starving to death. If the supplement does not contain FOS or GOS, the probiotic will likely die immediately.

However, even if the supplement contains a little FOS, the bacteria may only survive for a split-second longer. Without a hospitable environment—full of water, acidity and food—the bacteria will still die before reaching the intestines. A month to a bacteria colony is like a century in human time.

Imagine being placed in the desert with no water or food. We would likely die within just a few days. Even if we were given a meal on the first day, we would still die, although a day or two later than we would have without the meal. The hot blazing sun overhead, mercilessly beating down upon our bodies all day long would likely speed this process up a bit. This scenario might be comparable to taking unprotected probiotics on an empty stomach. Within an empty stomach, there are a number of enzymes and acids intended to kill off invading bacteria. While probiotic bacteria can and do live amongst acidic environments, the environment must have a particular pH and must also have food ready. For this reason, a hungry, empty stomach is not a hospitable environment for an unprotected probiotic.

One of the most protected environments for most lactobacilli and bifidobacteria is within dairy products. These bacteria love to ferment within diary environments. This is why they readily live within cow's milk, colostrum and breast milk. They are comfortable within the pH of milk. They also utilize lactose and the GOS and TOS that comes from it for food. This is why milk curdles so fast. Bacteria quickly expand their colonies within whole milk. They love this environment.

Fermbiotics

To assist probiotic survival when we take probiotic supplements, we should take them with dairy products or with other prebiotics if at all possible. Taking our probiotics with yogurt or kefir is even better, because these foods already come with a buffered acidic environment already prepared for new colony growth and plenty of nourishment—assuming the probiotic strains are not too competitive with each other.

This strategy of supplementing a probiotic together with its culture medium or fermentation natant, would appropriately called a fermbiotic. The ideal fermbiotic was one just described. Another possibility, however, comes from the commercial fermentation process. When supplemental probiotics are fermented in tanks, they are typically extracted and freeze-dried. When this takes place, the freeze-dried colony forming units are isolated and put into a caplet or capsule. A few manufacturers also harvest this fermentation substrate with the probiotic, and freeze-dry them together. Some have questioned whether this is enough substrate available to substantially assist probiotic growth.

Creating our own 'fermentation tanks' within our bodies offers the most assured strategy. Taking our probiotic supplement—whichever one we choose, together with a meal including fermented dairy products and FOS foods (say yogurt with bananas—yum) only makes sense.

Probiotic Foods

This naturally brings us to the subject of fermented or cultured foods. These can be fabulous sources for probiotics—already nicely cultured within a fermbiotic medium. These include yogurt and kefir, but also raw cheeses, traditional cottage cheese, traditional sour cream, traditional buttermilk, traditional sauerkraut, lassi, amasake (Japanese sweet rice drink), traditional miso, traditional tempeh, traditional tamari, traditional soy sauce and traditional kombucha tea and others.

Other foods utilize probiotics in their preparation. Traditional sourdough bread and bauerbrot are good examples. Most bread, in fact, uses some sort of (often probiotic) yeast fermentation process to prepare the flour for baking. In these, however, the probiotics are likely all killed during baking.

Some of the foods mentioned here are preceded by the word "traditional" because sadly, many of today's versions are pasteurized or otherwise acidified enough to kill any viable probiotic colonies. Both cottage cheese and butter were originally probiotic foods, for example, when we used to eat dairy products from our local dairies or own farms. Today, these two foods are produced commercially without probiotics. Ironically, even many commercial yogurts are unbelievably pasteurized prior to shipping—killing off most if not all of their viable colonies.

Another example is tamari and soy sauce. Today, most commercial versions are brewed with solvents. Probiotics are no longer part of these processes, as were the traditional versions.

For the sake of at least preserving the reputation of some of this rich tradition, here is a review of some of the more popular probiotic foods—and how they are (or were) made:

Traditional Yogurt

Because yogurt is usually produced using *L. bulgaricus, S. thermophilus* and sometimes *L. acidophilus*, it is certainly a good source of probiotics. However, we should clarify again that pasteurization kills many probiotics. This means that commercial yogurts that pasteurize the yogurt after it has been cultured will have killed most or all of those colonies used to convert the milk to yogurt. Some producers pasteurize the milk first and then make the yogurt. Still others add probiotics following pasteurization of the yogurt. These two methods are acceptable for gaining probiotic colonies—but not optimal. The best way to assure healthy probiotic colonies is to make fresh yogurt at home.

It is quite simple to make yogurt: After heating a pot of milk to 180 degrees F (82 C) momentarily, we can add a half-cup of starter (active yogurt from a previous batch or an active commercial yogurt) into the milk after it cools to about 105 degrees F (40 C). After stirring thoroughly, we can put the container in a warm, clean, dry place, with a clean towel or loose seal over the container. The mixture will sour and gel in about six to ten hours depending upon temperature. Then we can jar and refrigerate.

The ideal blend of probiotic species for a yogurt starter—one that was developed over the centuries by the Bulgarians—is a ratio of seven parts *S. thermophilus* to one part *L. bulgaricus.* This ratio produces the ideal sourness that is tasty yet tart. It also prevents the *L. bulgaricus* from outgrowing and overwhelming the *S. thermophilus.*

This later point is one of the reasons why yogurt starters that include *L. acidophilus* often fail to supply any *L. acidophilus* in the end product. *L. bulgaricus* is a hardy organism that will easily overtake *L. acidophilus* in a culture. The use of *L. acidophilus* in yogurt is not only wasteful, but possibly can result in an overly acidic flavor, as *L. bulgaricus* colonies swell with the lactic acid produced initially by *L. acidophilus*. In addition, it appears that *L. bulgaricus* produce small amounts of hydrogen peroxide—which knocks out the *L. acidophilus* colonies.

The moral of this also is not to expect much in the way of *L. acidophilus* in a commercial yogurt that blends *L. acidophilus* with *L. bulgaricus.*

Traditional Kefir

Kefir is a traditional drink originally developed in the Caucasus region of what is now considered southern Russia, Georgia, Armenia and Azerbaijan. Here Moslem tribe leaders vigorously protected their kefir recipe, as it was considered an esteemed and regal food with healing properties. The secret recipe was eventually ransomed by a young beautiful female Russian emissary who was kidnapped by a local prince. She wrestled a few kefir grains from the secrecy of the prince's family as a settlement for her abduction. She brought kefir into the Moscow market shortly thereafter and it spread as a highly prized healing food all over Russia and Europe. Kefir also became a focus of Soviet research, discovering some of the surprising benefits of probiotics we have outlined in this book.

Kefir uses fermented milk mixed with kefir grains that resemble little chunks of cauliflower. One tablespoon of kefir grains can be mixed with whole milk and sealed in a jar at room temperature. The milk is fermented overnight in a warm location with the starter grains. Depending upon the temperature, milk and kefir grains, it will take 1-3 days to completely ferment. The jar should be opened and swirled one to two times a day. The grains are screened or filtered out and utilized for the next batch. Cow's milk is most used, but sheep's milk, goat's milk or deer milk can also be used.

Buttermilk

Buttermilk is a soured beverage that was originally curdled from cream. Traditional buttermilk utilized the acids that probiotic bacteria produce for curdling. Today, forced curdling is done using commercially available acidic products. Cream of tartar, lemon juice or vinegar is added to heated and stirred whole milk at a rate of one tablespoon per cup of milk, until the curdling starts. After standing for 15 minutes and stirring another 15, it is refrigerated. See the butter section for the traditional method.

Traditional Butter

Today commercial butter contains no probiotics. Traditionally, butter was made with the cow's natural probiotics. The raw milk sits for a half-day or day depending upon temperature, until the cream rises to the top. The cream is taken from the milk to be churned and aged; letting the probiotics convert lactose to lactic acid. This creates a mix of buttermilk and butter. The buttermilk is strained off, leaving the butter. The butter can be further dried of moisture and mixed with salt for taste. Again, the probiotics from the raw milk will have matured the butter and buttermilk naturally.

Traditional Cottage Cheese

Commercial cottage cheese is now made without probiotics. It was a probiotic process before dairy processors began to pasteurize the product and force the curdling with lactic acids. Again, probiotics also produce the lactic acids that were used to curdle the product in traditional cottage cheese making. Skim milk with cream and buttermilk is probably the easiest way to make cottage cheese at home today, using the curds off the cream separation. The probiotics arising from the buttermilk help curdle the thickened milk and cream before separating the curds. Salt is one of the secrets to making a tasty cottage cheese.

Traditional Kimchi

Kimchi is a fermented cabbage with a wonderful history from Korea. Kimchi was considered a ceremonial food served to emperors and ambassadors. It also was highly regarded as a healing and tonic food. There are a variety of different recipes of kimchi, depending upon the region and occasion.

Kimchi can be made by slicing and mixing cabbage with warm water, salt, ginger, garlic, red pepper, green onions, oil and a crushed apple. It is then put into a sealed jar(s) at room temperature for 24 hours, before putting into the refrigerator to continue the fermenting process (*Lactobacillus kimchii* is a typical colonizer). After several weeks of continued fermentation in the fridge, it is ready for eating.

Traditional Miso

Miso is an ancient food from Japan. A well-made miso will contain over 160 strains of aerobic probiotic bacteria. This is because the ingredients are perfect prebiotics for these probiotics.

Miso is produced by fermenting beans and grains. Soybeans are often used, but other types of beans are also used. Equal parts soaked and cooked soybeans and rice are mixed. A fungi spore (koji, or *Aspergillus oryzae*) and salt is added to the rice prior to mixing. The mixture is put into a covered container in a dark, dry, room-temperature location and stirred occasionally. It can take up to a year of aging like this for the fermentation to result in a tasty miso.

When other beans other than soy are used, they will produce different varieties of miso. Shiromiso is white miso, kuromiso is black miso, and akamiso is red miso. They are each made with different beans. There are also various other miso recipies, many of which are highly guarded by their makers.

Traditional Shoyu

Shoyu is a traditional form of soy sauce made by blending a mixture of cooked soybeans and wheat, again with koji, or *Aspergillus oryzae*. The combination is fermented for an extended time. The aging process for shoyu is dependent upon the storage temperature and cooking methods used, and is also guarded.

Traditional Tempeh

Tempeh is an aged and fermented soybean food. It is extremely healthy and contains a combination of probiotics and naturally metabolized soy. Tempeh is made by first soaking dehulled soybeans for 10-12 hours. The beans are then cooked for 20 minutes and strained. The dry, cooked beans are then mixed with a tempeh starter containing *Rhyzopus oryzae, Rhizopus oligosporus* or both. The mixture is shaped and flattened (about a half-inch high) and put into a warm (room temperature) incubation container for a day or two. The cake will be full with white mycelium (fungal roots) when it is ready. It can then be eaten raw, baked, or toasted.

Other beans other than soy are also sometimes used to make tempeh. The trick is in getting good starter colonies.

Traditional Kombucha Tea

Kombucha tea is an ancient beverage from the orient. Its use dates back many centuries; and was used by China and Taiwanese emperors. Its use was later popularized in Russia, and then in Eastern Europe, where its reputation grew. A quality kombucha tea will contain a number of probiotics, including *Acetobacter xylinum, Acetobacter xylinoides, Glucobacter bluconicum, Acetobacter aceti, Saccharomycodes Ludwigii, Schizosaccharomyces pombe,* and

Picha fermentans—and other yeasts in the *Schizosaromyces* genus. The fermenting of these organisms renders a beverage that is full of nutrients and enzymes as well as healthy biotics. Kombucha has enjoyed a reputation of being detoxifying and revitalizing. Many alternative health experts have described it as a tonic.

Kombucha is made by blending a black or green tea with sugar, kombucha starter culture, and sometimes a bit of vinegar to create a slightly acidic environment. It is critical that a healthy starter be used. The mixture is then fermented in a warm, dry environment. It requires oxygen, yet will suffer from any toxins or bacteria from the air. Following a couple of weeks of fermentation, the product should be refrigerated to slow down growth and acidity.

Traditional Lassi

Lassi is a traditional and popular beverage from India—once enjoyed by kings and governors in ancient India. It is quite simple to make, as it is made with yogurt, fruit and spices. Quite simply, it is a blend of diluted yogurt with fruit pulp—often mango is used in the traditional lassi. A little salt, turmeric and sweetener give it a sweet-n-salty taste. Other spices are also sometimes used. Sugar is often added in today's versions, but honey and/or fruit are preferable.

Traditional Sauerkraut

Sauerkraut is a traditional German fermented food. It is made quite simply, by blending shredded cabbage and pickling salt (12:1, or 3 tablespoons of salt per five pounds of cabbage). The mixture is covered with water and put into a covered bowl or container. It is then stored in the dark in this semi-airtight cover for a month to two months at room temperature. Then it should be stored in the refrigerator in an enclosed container for a month or two to complete the fermentation of the cabbage. Probiotic bacteria such as *Lactobacillus plantarum* and *L. brevis* will typically overtake the early-growth bacteria during fermentation. This is a testament to the power of probiotics.

There are a number of other wonderful fermented foods that can be included into a probiotic-rich diet. This sampling illustrates the general techniques of fermentation. As we can see here, bacteria and fungi in our foods are not necessarily bad. To the contrary, if cultured correctly, they can be healthy for us, and may even help prevent infection from their more lethal cousins.

Threats to our Probiotics

How do we decimate healthy probiotic colonies? Very easily. In fact, many modern activities can threaten the survival of these precious populations.

Medications such as oral contraceptives, NSAIDS, corticosteroids, and many other chemical pharmaceuticals can kill off or shrink probiotic populations.

Antacids and acid-blockers in particular can threaten our probiotics because low HCL production opens the intestines to various pathobiotics. These competitive bacteria colonies can quickly reduce probiotic colonies. This possibly is increased with a pathobiotic-friendly diet. As invading bacteria begin to win over territory, probiotic populations can be dramatically decreased by pathobiotic colonies. The HCL content in the stomach is thus a critical gatekeeper for reducing pathobiotic populations.

A variety of manufactured chemicals added to foods, including preservatives and food color agents, also hamper the growth of probiotic populations. Preservatives, remember, are added to foods specifically to deter microbial growth and eliminate food spoilage. In the same way, preservatives will also retard our own probiotic bacteria populations.

As discussed earlier, without a balanced natural diet with plenty of plant-based foods, we will effectively starve or undernourish our probiotic populations. Foods lacking in fiber, high in trans-fats, high in refined sugar and/or low in nutrient content discourage probiotic growth. A diet high in animal proteins has been shown to decrease healthy flora as we have discussed. This is due to putrefaction. The slow movement of animal proteins through the digestive tract and the subsequent change in intestinal pH contribute to the overgrowth of pathogenic bacteria competitive to bifidobacteria and lactobacilli. As these bacteria decompose animal proteins, toxic amines such cadaverine and putrescine are produced. In addition to this, animal foods can introduce new pathobiotics into the system.

By far the worst enemies to healthy probiotic populations are antibiotic pharmaceuticals. A week's course of a pharmaceutical grade antibiotic can slaughter much of our viable probiotic colonies in one fell swoop. Imagine, not only killing off a current microbial infection, but also killing trillions of healthy probiotic colonies that have been attached to our intestines, colonizing for years if not decades.

We wonder why we have such a growing surge of autoimmune disease among western societies. As we are killing off our probiotics, we are killing off 70%-80% of our body's immune system. We are killing off our body's ability to digest food properly. The symbiotic relationship probiotics have with our body's immune system and digestive system evaporates, leaving these systems in disarray. This leaves our bodies open to an avalanche of infective microorganisms, digestive issues and autoimmune possibilities.

Unbelievably, this situation has been known to the cattle industry for many years. As cattlemen began dosing cattle with profuse amounts of antibiotics to keep crowded herds alive, cattle began dying of malnutrition and other diseases—even though they were eating enough. Because cattle can be cruelly slaughtered and examined immediately, it was not hard for veterinarians to discover that the lack of probiotics caused by the antibiotic dosing destroyed their ability to digest food and fight off other infections. This has led to a subsequent decrease in antibiotic dosing in the cattle industry, along with the popularity of probiotic supplementation for these animals. Even despite this, rigorous antibiotic dosing continues in an effort to keep cattle alive while being imprisoned in unhygienic feedlots where pathogenic (and mutating) bacteria congregate.

Effects of Stress and Sleep upon our Probiotics

Our balance and maintenance of probiotic colonies in our gut relates to not only what we consume, but also how we live. The evidence shows that probiotic colonies depend upon the nutritional content of our diet and our body's general internal environment. Just as we thrive off the food of the earth, and the cycles of the sun and weather, our probiotics depend upon regular body rhythms and low levels of stress.

An abundance of stress can lop off big numbers and stunt colony growth quite easily. Under stress, our vagus nerve will alter our flow of digestive juices. This alters the entire environment for intestinal probiotics. During anxiousness, our peristalsis wave rhythms will also change. They will pulse at different times, creating an unpredictable, uneasy environment. We might compare this situation to earthquake tremors that keep a population unnerved for days following a big quake.

Under stress, the digestive tract will not be given enough blood to carry nutrients and cycle toxins. Our digestive tract will slow in its mucous secretions and bile salts. This 'environmental crisis' will force our probiotic colonies to tolerate an increasingly inhospitable internal atmosphere.

Just as we stand comfortably on an earth that oscillates with rotational spin, magnetic fields and alternating weather currents, our probiotics thrive within the human body's oscillating nervous energy, thermal conditions, intestinal peristalsis, heart beat, oxygen flow and so many other rhythmic cycles.

Ulcers, intestinal polyps and an anxious, nervous demeanor, for example, might be compared to us living near an active volcano. The eruption of extra acidity or the bleeding of an ulcer or polyp could be lethal to the probiotics in that region, just as a volcanic eruption could decimate an entire city and population living nearby.

This all means that our probiotics have become connected to our stress levels. When we maintain low levels of stress, this is conducive to a thriving, healthy probiotic environment.

This conclusion is consistent with many studies that associate stress with many illnesses.

In addition, there are many clinical reports showing that opportunistic yeast and bacterial infections (candida and lyme disease, for example) immediately multiply following stressful episodes. This is consistent with the volumes of bacteria research, revealing that bacteria endeavor for survival and can easily recognize threats as well as opportunities for greater colonization. This is also consistent with the well-accepted quorum sensing abilities that bacteria colonies have, leading to communal responses to environmental cues.

The overgrowth of pathogenic bacteria and the destruction of probiotic bacteria during stressful times should point us towards the appropriate behavior when it comes to stress. Noting the undoubtedly conscious nature of these microorganisms, we must harmonize our activities with the needs of the populations of probiotic bacteria that dwell within in order to balance the activities of destructive bacteria. By offering a balanced environment for these creatures, they will thrive, and help our bodies thrive as well.

Various strategies can accomplish this. Obviously, we need to lower our external stressor levels. This means we avoid those situations that create stress. This means we slow down and relax. We try not to over-react to things. We try to reduce the amount of stress from noise, electromagnetic radiation levels, and confrontations with those around us.

This also means trying to establish and stick with regular eating and sleeping patterns. Going to bed around the same time, and eating around the same time every day will create a regular and comfortable internal environment for our probiotic friends.

There has been a lot of research done on sleep patterns, sleep stages, and the cycles between melatonin and cortisol that keep our bodies rhythmic. We know that when we sleep, our brain cells begin to process and 'download' information. During this period, our muscle cells and nerve cells enter into a recuperative state of rest and rejuvenation. We also know that without enough sleep, we get sick more frequently and die sooner.

What we may not realize is that our probiotics are hard at work when we are sleeping. When the body's stressors are lowered, they come into full bloom, and work to manage their local environments. This also means that they go into battle mode against pathogenic bacteria. They also stimulate the production of particular types of T-cells, B-cells and various cytokines. This is accomplished through the production of various chemical signals put out by probiotics, such as prolactin.

Our probiotics also respond to the swings between our melatonin and cortisol levels. During periods of high stress, our probiotics slow down. During periods of lower stress and sleep, our probiotics move into full swing. In other words, just as we cycle to the rhythms of light produced by the sun, our probiotics cycle to the rhythms produced by our energy and metabolic levels.

Stress creates a particular chemistry and flow of nutrients among every tissue system, including our digestive tract. When we are anxious, our vagus nerve is stimulated. Blood, oxygen and other nutrients are diverted from our intestines and stomach, and sent to the brain and muscles in preparation for our physical response to the stressor. This is why we will often have a "butterflies" sensation when we become stressed. The chemistry of the stomach and intestines has changed, and blood, oxygen, nutrients and mucous secretions are being diverted away from the digestive tract and into muscle tissues.

This basically starves our probiotic systems, and leaves them in an environment not conducive to growth.

Therefore, it is critical that we get enough good, sound sleep. Especially during periods of stress. When we are stressed, we need more sleep so that our probiotics can resume their normal activities.

If we are sleeping poorly, and our waking hours are filled with more stress, it is likely that our probiotic populations are under duress. For this reason, supplemental probiotics in therapeutic doses are suggested for periods of higher stress. These can assist in maintaining a healthy probiotic environment, assuming they are accompanied by healthy prebiotic foods. There is nothing like bringing in fresh troops when the current army has become stressed.

The Biotic Body

The vastness of the body's bacterial composition creates a renewed vision of the human anatomy. A thriving population of more than three trillion organisms renders a conclusion that our bodies have ten times more bacteria than cells. This resounding fact has led scientists to the concept of the microbiome—an "extended genome" of microorganism traits and genetics that better reflects our body's traits and pathology history than does our cellular DNA (Kinross, et al. 2006).

"Understanding the human microbiome may be as or more important to understanding human health than mapping and understanding the human genome," said Margaret McFall Ngai, Ph.D., microbiome researcher and professor of microbiology and immunology at University of Wisconsin's School of Medicine.

Certainly, our probiotic colonies lining just about every mucosal membrane and tissue system better predict future disease models. This conclusion is drawn from our creeping awareness that a predominance of disease pathologies is directly related to microbial imbalances among our living populations. Because our body's bacteria remember pathogens and adapt their antibiotic systems to those particular invaders, we can find within those adaptations a history of disease and immunity.

Actually, we may be far more connected to our resident probiotic colonies than ever suspected. While supplemented probiotics seem to be transients, the recent research that has indicated our lymphatic system may actually host genetic libraries and incubation chambers for our body's resident organisms has rocked our understanding of the human body.

As we've mentioned earlier, Duke University Medical Center researchers found evidence indicating that the vermiform appendix may actually be a "safe house" or library of incubated probiotic bacteria (Randal, *et al.* 2007). Their research indicated the appendix incubates and inoculates the intestines with specific strains of bacteria in response to pathogens.

This correlates well with strain research showing species isolated from the human gut mucosa implant more readily in the gut. These bacteria are keyed into their specific host.

The concept of the body housing and incubating resident bacteria may seem foreign even to medical experts, especially in the face of antibiotic use. Because other research has indicated that supplemented probiotics remain only a couple of weeks at the most after supplementation ceases, the growing assumption over the past decade among probiotic experts has been that our probiotic colonies are all transient in nature.

As we grasp this notion of our bodies being more bacterial than cellular, we come to a place where a healthy existence must be the result of conscious balance. We must balance not only our lifestyles, diets and activities: We must also coexist with the bacteria living around us and inside of us. We must be able to live with our bacteria—and strive to protect them as they strive to protect us.

Probiotic Consciousness

Cleve Backster's experiments (2003) over the last four decades with plants, cells and bacteria illustrated a unique cognition and communication process between these life forms and humans. Dr. Backster called this "primary perception."

Biologists have also found that bacteria mysteriously communicate perception throughout large colonies using a mechanicsm called "quorum sensing." This ability is now being seen among both probiotics and pathobiotics (Wu *et al.* 2009).

These understandings have also been confirmed by decades of focused research upon the ultraweak biophoton emission and cellular signalling led by Professor Fritz-Albert Popp from Germany's University of Marburg and several others. Professor Popp and associates referred to these communication mechanisms between bacteria and human cells as "low-level biological luminescence" (Chwirot and Popp 1991).

Professor Popp detected that microorganisms and cells produced weak levels of radiation that could be measured using sensitive equipment. The radiation was in the ultraviolet and visible spectrums—which classified the radiation as being light. He subsequently referred to this weak radiation as "biophotons." Furthermore, these types of radiation were observed during significant biological events—metabolic events that required coordinated efforts of many cells or colonies of microorganisms (Cohen and Popp 1997; others).

We know from many studies that bacteria respond to stimuli, avoid death, and avert pain. We know from medical research that bacteria will intelligently mutate and adapt to antibiotics. New antibiotic-resistant superbugs are examples of bacteria who have intelligently evaded death. Living bacteria also conduct all of the activities required for independent survival: eating, digesting, reproduction, movement, response to stimuli, sense perception, the intention to survive, and self-organization.

Research has also shown that colonies of specific probiotics are selective in their production of antibiotics and their stimulation of the immune system. We see specificity for reducing certain pathogens harmful to the body, such as *E. coli*, *Salmonella*, *Candida spp.* and others. This ability of probiotics to produce these selective effects illustrates not only consciousness, but also intelligence.

These and many other studies have confirmed that bacteria—whether pathogenic or probiotic—are conscious organisms, each maintaining intelligence, memory, and a desire to survive.

Our physical bodies, down to every cell, are also able to selectively identify, focus and respond to particular bacteria, viruses, cells and toxins with specificity, intelligence, memory, and appropriateness. The immune system's cells and proteins can somehow single out invaders among an environment containing trillions of microorganisms.

Certainly, there must an explanation for that fact that probiotics stimulate unique immune responses in different diseased states. How do they know what diseases are attacking the body?

Furthermore, there must be an explanation for the fact that supplemented probiotics exit the intestines in an orderly fashion within 10-14 days following supplementation. Could it be that our resident strains are repopulating their environment? Or could the immune system be rejecting these transients?

While a combination of these seems feasible, we cannot discount the possibility that those supplemented strains are also realizing, through subtle communications, that this body is not their permanent host. Perhaps this communication originates from our resident strains. Perhaps the communication arises from our immune system. Perhaps it is genetically programmed from within the transient bacteria.

Perhaps a combination of these intelligent processes is taking place. These questions, of course, require deeper realms of understanding and considerable research. Through deduction and current research data, we can at least conclude that some kind of intelligent communications are taking place between our immune systems and our tiny probiotic friends.

This is not that unreasonable. Consider the research data on immune system communications. Cytokine signalling, helper T-cell memorization, immunoglobulin programming and other immune system mechanisms all require signalling and communications. Bacteria communications involving bioluminescence and quorum sensing do not seem so abstract in comparison. Regardless of the names we give them, we know there are subtle yet powerful mechanisms of sensory reception and communication taking place between resident probiotics, supplemented probiotics, and our immune system.

Research now tells us that we can connect every cell of our body via common DNA expression: genetics and epigenetics. Though paracrine, juxtacrine and endocrine signalling we find organizational communication processes among cells. How do independent bacteria cooperate so well with the needs of the body? Bacteria DNA is certainly different from our DNA. Yet bacteria still have many of the same communication methods our cells have in terms of intercellular communication. A bacterium also has individuality and consciousness. From the research we've reviewed in this book, certainly we can agree that intelligent communications are taking place between our probiotics and our body's cells.

Our conclusion is found within the complexities of consciousness and survival. Just as we learn to adapt and (hopefully) act on behalf of our planet after recognizing environmental signs of stress (such as global warming), our probiotics can sense our body's environment, and respond appropriately to disease. Through their signalling mechanisms, they can construct and communicate common strategies to repel invaders and assist in the process of healing. This is the result of a conscious intent to survive. Humans have many of the same mechanisms, as we use radio and television signals to broadcast news and information, enabling us to enhance our possibilities for survival.

Our probiotic friends may be independent organisms, but they join us in our intent to survive. Just as we have choices about how we conduct ourselves within the larger biosphere of the planet earth, we also have choices about how we maintain the balance of the inner biosphere within each of our bodies.

Just as we are at a critical crossroads regarding the health of the planet, we are at a crossroads relating to our approach to the health of our bodies. The conscious approach respects the balances that exist within each of these two ecologies. The ignorant approach endangers both ecologies simultaneously.

Let's hope we choose the conscious approach in both regards.

References and Bibliography

Adoga AS, Otene AA, Yiltok SJ, Adekwu A, Nwaorgu OG. Cervical necrotizing fasciitis: case series and review of literature. *Niger J Med.* 2009 Apr-Jun;18(2):203-7.

Agarwal KN, Bhasin SK, Faridi MM, Mathur M, Gupta S. *Lactobacillus casei* in the control of acute diarrhea—a pilot study. *Indian Pediatr.* 2001 Aug;38(8):905-10.

Agerholm-Larsen L, Raben A, Haulrik N, Hansen AS, Manders M, Astrup A. Effect of 8 week intake of probiotic milk products on risk factors for cardiovascular diseases. *Eur J Clin Nutr.* 2000 Apr;54(4):288-97.

Agustina R, Lukito W, Firmansyah A, Suhardjo HN, Murniati D, Bindels J. The effect of early nutritional supplementation with a mixture of probiotic, prebiotic, fiber and micronutrients in infants with acute diarrhea in Indonesia. *Asia Pac J Clin Nutr.* 2007;16(3):435-42.

Ahmed M, Prasad J, Gill H, Stevenson L, Gopal P. Impact of consumption of different levels of *Bifidobacterium lactis* HN019 on the intestinal microflora of elderly human subjects. *J Nutr Health Aging.* 2007 Jan-Feb;11(1):26-31.

Ahmed, AA, McCarthy RD, Porter GA. Effect of milk constituents on hepatic cholesterogenesis. *Atherosclerosis.* 1979;32:347-57.

Ahola AJ, Yli-Knuuttila H, Suomalainen T, Poussa T, Ahlström A, Meurman JH, Korpela R. Short-term consumption of probiotic-containing cheese and its effect on dental caries risk factors. *Arch Oral Biol.* 2002 Nov;47(11):799-804.

Aihara K, Kajimoto O, Hirata H, Takahashi R, Nakamura Y. Effect of powdered fermented milk with *Lactobacillus helveticus* on subjects with high-normal blood pressure or mild hypertension. *J Am Coll Nutr.* 2005 Aug;24(4):257-65.

Akil I, Yilmaz O, Kurutepe S, Degerli K, Kavukcu S. Influence of oral intake of *Saccharomyces boulardii* on *Escherichia coli* in enteric flora. *Pediatr Nephrol.* 2006 Jun;21(6):807-10.

Allen SJ, Okoko B, Martinez E, Gregorio G, Dans LF. Probiotics for treating infectious diarrhea. *The Cochrane Library.* 2004;3. Chichester, UK: John Wiley & Sons, Ltd.

Amenta M, Cascio MT, Di Fiore P, Venturini I. Diet and chronic constipation. Benefits of oral supplementation with symbiotic zir fos (*Bifidobacterium longum* W11 + FOS Actilight). *Acta Biomed.* 2006 Dec;77(3):157-62.

Anderson JW, Gilliland SE. Effect of fermented milk (yogurt) containing *Lactobacillus acidophilus* L1 on serum cholesterol in hypercholesterolemic humans. *J Am Coll Nutr.* 1999 Feb;18(1):43-50.

Anukam K, Osazuwa E, Ahonkhai I, Ngwu M, Osemene G, Bruce AW, Reid G. Augmentation of antimicrobial metronidazole therapy of bacterial vaginosis with oral probiotic *Lactobacillus rhamnosus* GR-1 and *Lactobacillus reuteri* RC-14: randomized, double-blind, placebo controlled trial. *Microbes Infect.* 2006 May;8(6):1450-4.

Anukam KC, Osazuwa E, Osemene GI, Ehigiagbe F, Bruce AW, Reid G. Clinical study comparing probiotic Lactobacillus GR-1 and RC-14 with metronidazole vaginal gel to treat symptomatic bacterial vaginosis. *Microbes Infect.* 2006 Oct;8(12-13):2772-6.

Anukam KC, Osazuwa EO, Osadolor HB, Bruce AW, Reid G. Yogurt containing probiotic *Lactobacillus rhamnosus* GR-1 and *L. reuteri* RC-14 helps resolve moderate diarrhea and increases CD4 count in HIV/AIDS patients. *J Clin Gastroenterol.* 2008 Mar;42(3):239-43.

Araki K, Shinozaki T, Irie Y, Miyazawa Y. Trial of oral administration of *Bifidobacterium breve* for the prevention of rotavirus infections. *Kansenshogaku Zasshi.* 1999 Apr;73(4):305-10.

Armstrong BK. Absorption of vitamin B12 from the human colon. *Am J Clin Nutr.* 1968;21:298-9.

Armuzzi A, Cremonini F, Bartolozzi F, Canducci F, Candelli M, Ojetti V, Cammarota G, Anti M, De Lorenzo A, Pola P, Gasbarrini G, Gasbarrini A. The effect of oral administration of Lactobacillus GG on antibiotic-associated gastrointestinal side-effects during Helicobacter pylori eradication therapy. *Aliment Pharmacol Ther.* 2001 Feb;15(2):163-9.

Arrigo G, D'Angelo A. Achromycin and anaphylactic shock. *Riv Patol Clin.* 1959 Oct;14:719-22.

Arunachalam K, Gill HS, Chandra RK. Enhancement of natural immune function by dietary consumption of *Bifidobacterium lactis* (HN019). *Eur J Clin Nutr.* 2000 Mar;54(3):263-7.

Arvola T, Laiho K, Torkkeli S, Mykkänen H, Salminen S, Maunula L, Isolauri E. Prophylactic Lactobacillus GG reduces antibiotic-associated diarrhea in children with respiratory infections: a randomized study. *Pediatrics.* 1999 Nov;104(5):e64.

Aso Y, Akaza H, Kotake T, Tsukamoto T, Imai K, Naito S. Preventive effect of a *Lactobacillus casei* preparation on the recurrence of superficial bladder cancer in a double-blind trial. The BLP Study Group. *Eur Urol.* 1995;27(2):104-9.

Aso Y, Akazan H. Prophylactic effect of a *Lactobacillus casei* preparation on the recurrence of superficial bladder cancer. BLP Study Group. *Urol Int.* 1992;49(3):125-9.

Ataie-Jafari A, Larijani B, Alavi Majd H, Tahbaz F. Cholesterol-lowering effect of probiotic yogurt in comparison with ordinary yogurt in mildly to moderately hypercholesterolemic subjects. *Ann Nutr Metab.* 2009;54(1):22-7.

259

Backster C. *Primary Perception: Biocommunication with Plants, Living Foods, and Human Cells.* Anza, CA: White Rose Millennium Press, 2003.

Bai AP, Ouyang Q, Xiao XR, Li SF. Probiotics modulate inflammatory cytokine secretion from inflamed mucosa in active ulcerative colitis. *Int J Clin Pract.* 2006 Mar;60(3):284-8.

Baik HW. Nutritional therapy in gastrointestinal disease. *Korean J Gastroenterol.* 2004 Jun;43(6):331-40.

Baker SM. *Detoxification and Healing.* Chicago: Contemporary Books, 2004.

Balimane P, Yong-Haen H, Chong S. Current Industrial Practices of Assessing Permeability and P-Glycoprotein Interaction. *J AAPS* 2006; 8(1).

Ballentine R. *Diet & Nutrition: A holistic approach.* Honesdale, PA: Himalayan Int., 1978.

Ballentine RM. *Radical Healing.* New York: Harmony Books, 1999.

Balli F, Bertolani P, Giberti G, Amarri S. High-dose oral bacteria-therapy for chronic non-specific diarrhea of infancy. *Pediatr Med Chir.* 1992 Jan-Feb;14(1):13-5.

Baron M. A patented strain of Bacillus coagulans increased immune response to viral challenge. *Postgrad Med.* 2009 Mar;121(2):114-8.

Bartram HP, Scheppach W, Gerlach S, Ruckdeschel G, Kelber E, Kasper H. Does yogurt enriched with *Bifidobacterium longum* affect colonic microbiology and fecal metabolites in health subjects? *Am J Clin Nutr.* 1994 Feb;59(2):428-32.

Batmanghelidj F. *Your Body's Many Cries for Water.* 2nd Ed. Vienna, VA: Global Health, 1997.

Basu S, Chatterjee M, Ganguly S, Chandra PK. Effect of *Lactobacillus rhamnosus* GG in persistent diarrhea in Indian children: a randomized controlled trial. *J Clin Gastroenterol.* 2007 Sep;41(8):756-60.

Basu S, Chatterjee M, Ganguly S, Chandra PK. Efficacy of *Lactobacillus rhamnosus* GG in acute watery diarrhoea of Indian children: a randomised controlled trial. *J Paediatr Child Health.* 2007 Dec;43(12):837-42.

Beausoleil M, Fortier N, Guénette S, L'ecuyer A, Savoie M, Franco M, Lachaine J, Weiss K. Effect of a fermented milk combining *Lactobacillus acidophilus* Cl1285 and *Lactobacillus casei* in the prevention of antibiotic-associated diarrhea: a randomized, double-blind, placebo-controlled trial. *Can J Gastroenterol.* 2007 Nov;21(11):732-6.

Bengmark S. Immunonutrition: role of biosurfactants, fiber, and probiotic bacteria. *Nutrition.* 1998 Jul-Aug;14(7-8):585-94.

Billoo AG, Memon MA, Khaskheli SA, Murtaza G, Iqbal K, Saeed Shekhani M, Siddiqi AQ. Role of a probiotic (*Saccharomyces boulardii*) in management and prevention of diarrhoea. *World J Gastroenterol.* 2006 Jul 28;12(28):4557-60.

Bin-Nun A, Bromiker R, Wilschanski M, Kaplan M, Rudensky B, Caplan M, Hammerman C. Oral probiotics prevent necrotizing enterocolitis in very low birth weight neonates. *J Pediatr.* 2005 Aug;147(2):192-6.

Bliakher MS, Fedorova IM, Lopatina TK, Arkhipov SN, Kapustin IV, Ramazanova ZK, Karpova NV, Ivanov VA, Sharapov NV. Acilact and improvement of the health status of sickly children. *Vestn Ross Akad Med Nauk.* 2005;(12):32-5.

Bode C, Bode JC. Effect of alcohol consumption on the gut. *Best Pract Res Clin Gastroenterol.* 2003 Aug;17(4):575-92.

Boivin DB, Czeisler CA. Resetting of circadian melatonin and cortisol rhythms in humans by ordinary room light. *Neuroreport.* 1998 Mar 30;9(5):779-82.

Boivin DB, Duffy JF, Kronauer RE, Czeisler CA. Dose-response relationships for resetting of human circadian clock by light. *Nature.* 1996 Feb 8;379(6565):540-2.

Bongaerts GP, Severijnen RS. Preventive and curative effects of probiotics in atopic patients. *Med Hypotheses.* 2005;64(6):1089-92.

Böttcher MF, Abrahamsson TR, Fredriksson M, Jakobsson T, Björkstén B. Low breast milk TGF-beta2 is induced by *Lactobacillus reuteri* supplementation and associates with reduced risk of sensitization during infancy. *Pediatr Allergy Immunol.* 2008 Sep;19(6):497-504.

Boylan R, Li Y, Simeonova L, Sherwin G, Kreisman J, Craig RG, Ship JA, McCutcheon JA. Reduction in bacterial contamination of toothbrushes using the Violight ultraviolet light activated toothbrush sanitizer. *Am J Dent.* 2008 Oct;21(5):313-7.

Brasseur JG, Nicosia MA, Pal A, Miller LS. Function of longitudinal vs circular muscle fibers in esophageal peristalsis, deduced with mathematical modeling. *World J Gastroenterol.* 2007 Mar 7;13(9):1335-46.

Bu LN, Chang MH, Ni YH, Chen HL, Cheng CC. *Lactobacillus casei* rhamnosus Lcr35 in children with chronic constipation. *Pediatr Int.* 2007 Aug;49(4):485-90.

Caglar E, Cildir SK, Ergeneli S, Sandalli N, Twetman S. Salivary mutans streptococci and lactobacilli levels after ingestion of the probiotic bacterium *Lactobacillus reuteri* ATCC 55730 by straws or tablets. *Acta Odontol Scand.* 2006 Oct;64(5):314-8.

Caglar E, Kavaloglu SC, Kuscu OO, Sandalli N, Holgerson PL, Twetman S. Effect of chewing gums containing xylitol or probiotic bacteria on salivary mutans streptococci and lactobacilli. *Clin Oral Investig.* 2007 Dec;11(4):425-9.

REFERENCES AND BIBLIOGRAPHY

Caglar E, Kuscu OO, Cildir SK, Kuvvetli SS, Sandalli N. A probiotic lozenge administered medical device and its effect on salivary mutans streptococci and lactobacilli. *Int J Paediatr Dent.* 2008 Jan;18(1):35-9.

Caglar E, Kuscu OO, Selvi Kuvvetli S, Kavaloglu Cildir S, Sandalli N, Twetman S. Short-term effect of ice-cream containing *Bifidobacterium lactis* Bb-12 on the number of salivary mutans streptococci and lacto-bacilli. *Acta Odontol Scand.* 2008 Jun;66(3):154-8.

Campieri C, Campieri M, Bertuzzi V, Swennen E, Matteuzzi D, Stefoni S, Pirovano F, Centi C, Ulisse S, Famularo G, De Simone C. Reduction of oxaluria after an oral course of lactic acid bacteria at high concentration. *Kidney Int.* 2001 Sep;60(3):1097-105.

Canani RB, Cirillo P, Terrin G, Cesarano L, Spagnuolo MI, De Vincenzo A, Albano F, Passariello A, De Marco G, Manguso F, Guarino A. Probiotics for treatment of acute diarrhoea in children: randomised clinical trial of five different preparations. *BMJ.* 2007 Aug 18;335(7615):340.

Canducci F, Armuzzi A, Cremonini F, Cammarota G, Bartolozzi F, Pola P, Gasbarrini G, Gasbarrini A. A lyophilized and inactivated culture of *Lactobacillus acidophilus* increases Helicobacter pylori eradication rates. *Aliment Pharmacol Ther.* 2000 Dec;14(12):1625-9.

Canducci F, Cremonini F, Armuzzi A, Di Caro S, Gabrielli M, Santarelli L, Nista E, Lupascu A, De Martini D, Gasbarrini A. Probiotics and Helicobacter pylori eradication. *Dig Liver Dis.* 2002 Sep;34 Suppl 2:S81-3.

Carpita N. C., Kanabus J., Housley T. L. Linkage structure of fructans and fructan oligomers from Triticum aestivum and Festuca arundinacea leaves. *J. Plant Physiol.* 1989;134:162-168

Cats A, Kuipers EJ, Bosschaert MA, Pot RG, Vandenbroucke-Grauls CM, Kusters JG. Effect of frequent consumption of a *Lactobacillus casei*-containing milk drink in Helicobacter pylori-colonized subjects. *Aliment Pharmacol Ther.* 2003 Feb;17(3):429-35.

Chaitow L, Trenev N. *Probiotics: The revolutionary, 'friendly bacteria way to vital health and well-being.* New York: Thorsons, 1990.

Chao A, Thun MJ, Connell CJ, McCullough ML, Jacobs EJ, Flanders WD, Rodriguez C, Sinha R, Calle EE. Meat consumption and risk of colorectal cancer. *JAMA.* 2005 Jan 12;293(2):172-82.

Chapat L, Chemin K, Dubois B, Bourdet-Sicard R, Kaiserlian D. Lactobacillus casei reduces CD8+ T cell-mediated skin inflammation. *Eur J Immunol.* 2004 Sep;34(9):2520-8.

Chiang BL, Sheih YH, Wang LH, Liao CK, Gill HS. Enhancing immunity by dietary consumption of a probiotic lactic acid bacterium (*Bifidobacterium lactis* HN019): optimization and definition of cellular immune responses. *Eur J Clin Nutr.* 2000 Nov;54(11):849-55.

Chilton F, Tucker L. *Win the War Within.* New York: Rodale, 2006.

Chouraqui JP, Grathwohl D, Labaune JM, Hascoet JM, de Montgolfier I, Leclaire M, Giarre M, Steenhout P. Assessment of the safety, tolerance, and protective effect against diarrhea of infant formulas containing mixtures of probiotics or probiotics and prebiotics in a randomized controlled trial. *Am J Clin Nutr.* 2008 May;87(5):1365-73.

Chouraqui JP, Van Egroo LD, Fichot MC. Acidified milk formula supplemented with *Bifidobacterium lactis*: impact on infant diarrhea in residential care settings. *J Pediatr Gastroenterol Nutr.* 2004 Mar;38(3):288-92.

Chwirot WB, Popp F. White-light-induced luminescence and mitotic activity of yeast cells. *Folia Histochemica et Cytobiologica.* 1991;29(4):155.

Cianci A, Giordano R, Delia A, Grasso E, Amodeo A, De Leo V, Caccamo F. Efficacy of *Lactobacillus rhamnosus* GR-1 and of *Lactobacillus reuteri* RC-14 in the treatment and prevention of vaginoses and bacterial vaginitis relapses. *Minerva Ginecol.* 2008 Oct;60(5):369-76.

Clerici M, Balotta C, Meroni L, Ferrario E, Riva C, Trabattoni D, Ridolfo A,Villa M, Shearer GM, Moroni M, Galli M. Type 1 cytokine production and low prevalence of viral isolation correlate with long-term nonprogression in HIV infection. *AIDS Res Hum Retroviruses.* 1996 Jul 20;12(11):1053-61.

Cobo Sanz JM, Mateos JA, Muñoz Conejo A. Effect of *Lactobacillus casei* on the incidence of infectious conditions in children. *Nutr Hosp.* 2006 Jul-Aug;21(4):547-51.

Cohen S, Popp F. Biophoton emission of the human body. *J Photochem & Photobio.* 1997;B 40:187-189.

Colecchia A, Vestito A, La Rocca A, Pasqui F, Nikiforaki A, Festi D; Symbiotic Study Group. Effect of a symbiotic preparation on the clinical manifestations of irritable bowel syndrome, constipation-variant. Results of an open, uncontrolled multicenter study. *Minerva Gastroenterol Dietol.* 2006 Dec;52(4):349-58.

Colodner R, Edelstein H, Chazan B, Raz R. Vaginal colonization by orally administered *Lactobacillus rhamnosus* GG. *Isr Med Assoc J.* 2003 Nov;5(11):767-9.

Consumer Reports. Probiotics: Are enough in your diet? *Cons Rpts Mag.* 2005:34-35.

Conway PL, Gorbach SL, Goldin BR. Survival of lactic acid bacteria in the human stomach and adhesion to intestinal cells. *J Dairy Sci.* 1987 Jan;70(1):1-12.

Corrêa NB, Péret Filho LA, Penna FJ, Lima FM, Nicoli JR. A randomized formula controlled trial of *Bifidobacterium lactis* and *Streptococcus thermophilus* for prevention of antibiotic-associated diarrhea in infants. *J Clin Gastroenterol.* 2005 May-Jun;39(5):385-9.

Dalaly BK, Eitenmiller RR, Friend BA, Shahani KM. Human milk ribonuclease. *Biochim Biophys Acta.* 1980 Oct;615(2):381-91.

Dalaly BK, Eitenmiller RR, Vakil JR, Shahani KM. Simultaneous isolation of human milk ribonuclease and lysozyme. Anal Biochem. 1970 Sep;37(1):208-11.

De Preter V, Raemen H, Cloetens L, Houben E, Rutgeerts P, Verbeke K. Effect of dietary intervention with different pre- and probiotics on intestinal bacterial enzyme activities. *Eur J Clin Nutr.* 2008 Feb;62(2):225-31.

De Simone C, Ciardi A, Grassi A, Lambert Gardini S, Tzantzoglou S, Trinchieri V, Moretti S, Jirillo E. Effect of *Bifidobacterium bifidum* and *Lactobacillus acidophilus* on gut mucosa and peripheral blood B lymphocytes. *Immunopharmacol Immunotoxicol.* 1992;14(1-2):331-40.

de Vrese M, Rautenberg P, Laue C, Koopmans M, Herremans T, Schrezenmeir J. Probiotic bacteria stimulate virus-specific neutralizing antibodies following a booster polio vaccination. *Eur J Nutr.* 2005 Oct;44(7):406-13.

de Vrese M, Winkler P, Rautenberg P, Harder T, Noah C, Laue C, Ott S, Hampe J, Schreiber S, Heller K, Schrezenmeir J. Effect of *Lactobacillus gasseri* PA 16/8, *Bifidobacterium longum* SP 07/3, *B. bifidum* MF 20/5 on common cold episodes: a double blind, randomized, controlled trial. *Clin Nutr.* 2005 Aug;24(4):481-91.

Dean C. *Death by Modern Medicine.* Belleville, ON: Matrix Verite-Media, 2005.

Delia A, Morgante G, Rago G, Musacchio MC, Petraglia F, De Leo V. Effectiveness of oral administration of Lactobacillus paracasei subsp. paracasei F19 in association with vaginal suppositories of Lactobacillus acidofilus in the treatment of vaginosis and in the prevention of recurrent vaginitis. *Minerva Ginecol.* 2006 Jun;58(3):227-31.

DeMan, JC, Rogosa M, Sharpe ME. A medium for the cultivation of lactobacilli. *J Bacteriol.* 1960:23;130.

Denys GA, Koch KM, Dowzicky MJ. Distribution of resistant gram-positive organisms across the census regions of the United States and in vitro activity of tigecycline, a new glycylcycline antimicrobial. *Am J Infect Control.* 2007 Oct;35(8):521-6.

Depeint F, Tzortzis G, Vulevic J, I'anson K, Gibson GR. Prebiotic evaluation of a novel galactooligosaccharide mixture produced by the enzymatic activity of *Bifidobacterium bifidum* NCIMB 41171, in healthy humans: a randomized, double-blind, crossover, placebo-controlled intervention study. *Am J Clin Nutr.* 2008 Mar;87(3):785-91.

Desbonnet L, Garrett L, Clarke G, Bienenstock J, Dinan TG. The probiotic Bifidobacteria infantis: An assessment of potential antidepressant properties in the rat. *J Psychiatr Res.* 2008 Dec;43(2):164-74.

DeWitt RC, Kudsk KA. The gut's role in metabolism, mucosal barrier function, and gut immunology. *Infect Dis Clin North Am.* 1999 Jun;13(2):465-81.

Di Marzio L, Centi C, Cinque B, Masci S, Giuliani M, Arcieri A, Zicari L, De Simone C, Cifone MG. Effect of the lactic acid bacterium *Streptococcus thermophilus* on stratum corneum ceramide levels and signs and symptoms of atopic dermatitis patients. *Exp Dermatol.* 2003 Oct;12(5):615-20.

Dierksen KP, Moore CJ, Inglis M, Wescombe PA, Tagg JR. The effect of ingestion of milk supplemented with salivaricin A-producing Streptococcus salivarius on the bacteriocin-like inhibitory activity of streptococcal populations on the tongue. *FEMS Microbiol Ecol.* 2007 Mar;59(3):584-91.

Dimitonova SP, Danova ST, Serkedjieva JP, Bakalov BV. Antimicrobial activity and protective properties of vaginal lactobacilli from healthy Bulgarian women. *Anaerobe.* 2007 Oct-Dec;13(5-6):178-84.

Dinleyici EC, Eren M, Yargic ZA, Dogan N, Vandenplas Y. Clinical efficacy of *Saccharomyces boulardii* and metronidazole compared to metronidazole alone in children with acute bloody diarrhea caused by amebiasis: a prospective, randomized, open label study. *Am J Trop Med Hyg.* 2009 Jun;80(6):953-5.

Diop L, Guillou S, Durand H. Probiotic food supplement reduces stress-induced gastrointestinal symptoms in volunteers: a double-blind, placebo-controlled, randomized trial. *Nutr Res.* 2008 Jan;28(1):1-5.

Dotolo Institute. *The Study of Colon Hydrotherapy.* Pinellas Park, FL: Dotolo, 2003.

Drago L, De Vecchi E, Nicola L, Zucchetti E, Gismondo MR, Vicariotto F. Activity of a *Lactobacillus acidophilus*-based douche for the treatment of bacterial vaginosis. *J Altern Complement Med.* 2007 May;13(4):435-8.

Drouault-Holowacz S, Bieuvelet S, Burckel A, Cazaubiel M, Dray X, Marteau P. A double blind randomized controlled trial of a probiotic combination in 100 patients with irritable bowel syndrome. *Gastroenterol Clin Biol.* 2008 Feb;32(2):147-52.

Elmer GW, McFarland LV, Surawicz CM, Danko L, Greenberg RN. Behaviour of *Saccharomyces boulardii* in recurrent *Clostridium difficile* disease patients. *Aliment Pharmacol Ther.* 1999 Dec;13(12):1663-8.

Fabian E, Elmadfa I. Influence of daily consumption of probiotic and conventional yoghurt on the plasma lipid profile in young healthy women. *Ann Nutr Metab.* 2006;50(4):387-93.

Fabian E, Majchrzak D, Dieminger B, Meyer E, Elmadfa I. Influence of probiotic and conventional yoghurt on the status of vitamins B1, B2 and B6 in young healthy women. *Ann Nutr Metab.* 2008;52(1):29-36.

Fang H, Elina T, Heikki A, Seppo S. Modulation of humoral immune response through probiotic intake. *FEMS Immunol Med Microbiol.* 2000 Sep;29(1):47-52.

Fanigliulo L, Comparato G, Aragona G, Cavallaro L, Iori V, Maino M, Cavestro GM, Soliani P, Sianesi M, Franzè A, Di Mario F. Role of gut microflora and probiotic effects in the irritable bowel syndrome. *Acta Biomed.* 2006 Aug;77(2):85-9.

Farber JE, Ross J, Stephens G. Antibiotic anaphylaxis. *Calif Med.* 1954 Jul;81(1):9-11.

Farber JE, Ross J. Antibiotic anaphylaxis; a note on the treatment and prevention of severe reactions to penicillin, streptomycin and dihydrostreptomycin. *Med Times.* 1952 Jan;80(1):28-30.

Fasano A, Shea-Donohue T. Mechanisms of disease: the role of intestinal barrier function in the pathogenesis of gastrointestinal autoimmune diseases. *Nat Clin Pract Gastroenterol Hepatol.* 2005 Sep;2(9):416-22.

Felley CP, Corthésy-Theulaz I, Rivero JL, Sipponen P, Kaufmann M, Bauerfeind P, Wiesel PH, Brassart D, Pfeifer A, Blum AL, Michetti P. Favourable effect of an acidified milk (LC-1) on *Helicobacter pylori* gastritis in man. *Eur J Gastroenterol Hepatol.* 2001 Jan;13(1):25-9.

Ferencík M, Ebringer L, Mikes Z, Jahnová E, Ciznár I. Successful modification of human intestinal microflora with oral administration of lactic acid bacteria. *Bratisl Lek Listy.* 1999 May;100(5):238-45.

Ferrier L, Berard F, Debrauwer L, Chabo C, Langella P, Bueno L, Fioramonti J. Impairment of the intestinal barrier by ethanol involves enteric microflora and mast cell activation in rodents. *Am J Pathol.* 2006 Apr;168(4):1148-54.

Firmesse O, Alvaro E, Mogenet A, Bresson JL, Lemée R, Le Ruyet P, Bonhomme C, Lambert D, Andrieux C, Doré J, Corthier G, Furet JP, Rigottier-Gois L. Fate and effects of Camembert cheese microorganisms in the human colonic microbiota of healthy volunteers after regular Camembert consumption. *Int J Food Microbiol.* 2008 Jul 15;125(2):176-81.

Forestier C, Guelon D, Cluytens V, Gillart T, Sirot J, De Champs C. Oral probiotic and prevention of Pseudomonas aeruginosa infections: a randomized, double-blind, placebo-controlled pilot study in intensive care unit patients. *Crit Care.* 2008;12(3):R69.

Francavilla R, Lionetti E, Castellaneta SP, Magistà AM, Maurogiovanni G, Bucci N, De Canio A, Indrio F, Cavallo L, Ierardi E, Miniello VL. Inhibition of *Helicobacter pylori* infection in humans by *Lactobacillus reuteri* ATCC 55730 and effect on eradication therapy: a pilot study. *Helicobacter.* 2008 Apr;13(2):127-34.

Friend BA, Shahani KM, Long CA, Vaughn LA. The effect of processing and storage on key enzymes, B vitamins, and lipids of mature human milk. Evaluation of fresh samples and effects of freezing and frozen storage. *Pediatr Res.* 1983 Jan;17(1):61-4.

Friend BA, Shahani KM. Characterization and evaluation of Aspergillus oryzae lactase coupled to a regenerable support. *Biotechnol Bioeng.* 1982 Feb;24(2):329-45.

Fujii T, Ohtsuka Y, Lee T, Kudo T, Shoji H, Sato H, Nagata S, Shimizu T, Yamashiro Y. *Bifidobacterium breve* enhances transforming growth factor beta1 signaling by regulating Smad7 expression in preterm infants. *J Pediatr Gastroenterol Nutr.* 2006 Jul;43(1):83-8.

Fujimori S, Gudis K, Mitsui K, Seo T, Yonezawa M, Tanaka S, Tatsuguchi A, Sakamoto C. A randomized controlled trial on the efficacy of synbiotic versus probiotic or prebiotic treatment to improve the quality of life in patients with ulcerative colitis. *Nutrition.* 2009 May;25(5):520-5.

Furrie E, Macfarlane S, Kennedy A, Cummings JH, Walsh SV, O'neil DA, Macfarlane GT. Synbiotic therapy (*Bifidobacterium longum*/Synergy 1) initiates resolution of inflammation in patients with active ulcerative colitis: a randomised controlled pilot trial. *Gut.* 2005 Feb;54(2):242-9.

Gaón D, Doweck Y, Gómez Zavaglia A, Ruiz Holgado A, Oliver G. Lactose digestion by milk fermented with *Lactobacillus acidophilus* and *Lactobacillus casei* of human origin. *Medicina (B Aires).* 1995;55(3):237-42.

Gaón D, García H, Winter L, Rodríguez N, Quintás R, González SN, Oliver G. Effect of Lactobacillus strains and *Saccharomyces boulardii* on persistent diarrhea in children. *Medicina (B Aires).* 2003;63(4):293-8.

Gaón D, Garmendia C, Murrielo NO, de Cucco Games A, Cerchio A, Quintas R, González SN, Oliver G. Effect of Lactobacillus strains (*L. casei* and *L. Acidophilus* Strains cerela) on bacterial overgrowth-related chronic diarrhea. *Medicina.* 2002;62(2):159-63.

Garcia Vilela E, De Lourdes De Abreu Ferrari M, Oswaldo Da Gama Torres H, Guerra Pinto A, Carolina Carneiro Aguirre A, Paiva Martins F, Marcos Andrade Goulart E, Sales Da Cunha A. Influence of *Saccharomyces boulardii* on the intestinal permeability of patients with Crohn's disease in remission. *Scand J Gastroenterol.* 2008;43(7):842-8.

Gawrońska A, Dziechciarz P, Horvath A, Szajewska H. A randomized double-blind placebo-controlled trial of Lactobacillus GG for abdominal pain disorders in children. *Aliment Pharmacol Ther.* 2007 Jan 15;25(2):177-84.

Gill HS, Rutherfurd KJ, Cross ML, Gopal PK. Enhancement of immunity in the elderly by dietary supplementation with the probiotic *Bifidobacterium lactis* HN019. *Am J Clin Nutr.* 2001 Dec;74(6):833-9.

Gill HS, Rutherfurd KJ, Cross ML. Dietary probiotic supplementation enhances natural killer cell activity in the elderly: an investigation of age-related immunological changes. *J Clin Immunol.* 2001 Jul;21(4):264-71.

Gionchetti P, Rizzello F, Venturi A, Brigidi P, Matteuzzi D, Bazzocchi G, Poggioli G, Miglioli M, Campieri M. Oral bacteriotherapy as maintenance treatment in patients with chronic pouchitis: a double-blind, placebo-controlled trial. *Gastroenterology.* 2000 Aug;119(2):305-9.

Gittleman AL. *Guess What Came to Dinner.* New York: Avery, 2001.

Glück U, Gebbers J. Ingested probiotics reduce nasal colonization with pathogenic bacteria (*Staphylococcus aureus, Streptococcus pneumoniae*, and b-hemolytic streptococci. *Am J. Clin. Nutr.* 2003;77:517-520.

Goldin BR, Adlercreutz H, Gorbach SL, Warram JH, Dwyer JT, Swenson L, Woods MN. Estrogen excretion patterns and plasma levels in vegetarian and omnivorous women. *N Engl J Med.* 1982 Dec 16;307(25):1542-7.

Goldin BR, Swenson L, Dwyer J, Sexton M, Gorbach SL. Effect of diet and *Lactobacillus acidophilus* supplements on human fecal bacterial enzymes. *J Natl Cancer Inst.* 1980 Feb;64(2):255-61.

Goossens D, Jonkers D, Russel M, Stobberingh E, Van Den Bogaard A, StockbrUgger R. The effect of *Lactobacillus plantarum* 299v on the bacterial composition and metabolic activity in faeces of healthy volunteers: a placebo-controlled study on the onset and duration of effects. *Aliment Pharmacol Ther.* 2003 Sep 1;18(5):495-505.

Goossens DA, Jonkers DM, Russel MG, Stobberingh EE, Stockbrügger RW. The effect of a probiotic drink with *Lactobacillus plantarum* 299v on the bacterial composition in faeces and mucosal biopsies of rectum and ascending colon. *Aliment Pharmacol Ther.* 2006 Jan 15;23(2):255-63.

Gotteland M, Poliak L, Cruchet S, Brunser O. Effect of regular ingestion of *Saccharomyces boulardii* plus inulin or *Lactobacillus acidophilus* LB in children colonized by *Helicobacter pylori.* *Acta Paediatr.* 2005 Dec;94(12):1747-51.

Grasso F, Grillo C, Musumeci F, Triglia A, Rodolico G, Cammisuli F, Rinzivillo C, Fragati G, Santuccio A, Rodolico M. Photon emission from normal and tumour human tissues. *Experientia.* 1992;48:10-13.

Grönlund MM, Gueimonde M, Laitinen K, Kociubinski G, Grönroos T, Salminen S, Isolauri E. Maternal breast-milk and intestinal bifidobacteria guide the compositional development of the *Bifidobacterium* microbiota in infants at risk of allergic disease. *Clin Exp Allergy.* 2007 Dec;37(12):1764-72.

Groppo FC, Ramacciato JC, Simões RP, Flório FM, Sartoratto A. Antimicrobial activity of garlic, tea tree oil, and chlorhexidine against oral microorganisms. *Int Dent J.* 2002 Dec;52(6):433-7.

Guarino A, Canani RB, Spagnuolo MI, Albano F, Di Benedetto L. Oral bacterial therapy reduces the duration of symptoms and of viral excretion in children with mild diarrhea. *J Pediatr Gastroenterol Nutr.* 1997 Nov;25(5):516-9.

Guerin-Danan C, Chabanet C, Pedone C, Popot F, Vaissade P, Bouley C, Szylit O, Andrieux C. Milk fermented with yogurt cultures and *Lactobacillus casei* compared with yogurt and gelled milk: influence on intestinal microflora in healthy infants. *Am J Clin Nutr.* 1998 Jan;67(1):111-7.

Guslandi M, Giollo P, Testoni PA. A pilot trial of *Saccharomyces boulardii* in ulcerative colitis. *Eur J Gastroenterol Hepatol.* 2003 Jun;15(6):697-8.

Guslandi M, Mezzi G, Sorghi M, Testoni PA. *Saccharomyces boulardii* in maintenance treatment of Crohn's disease. *Dig Dis Sci.* 2000 Jul;45(7):1462-4.

Haarman M, Knol J. Quantitative real-time PCR assays to identify and quantify fecal *Bifidobacterium* species in infants receiving a prebiotic infant formula. *Appl Environ Microbiol.* 2005 May;71(5):2318-24.

Hallén A, Jarstrand C, Påhlson C. Treatment of bacterial vaginosis with lactobacilli. *Sex Transm Dis.* 1992 May-Jun;19(3):146-8.

Harris LA, Chang L. Irritable bowel syndrome: new and emerging therapies. *Curr Opin Gastroenterol.* 2006 Mar;22(2):128-35.

Harvey HP, Solomon HJ. Acute anaphylactic shock due to para-aminosalicylic acid. *Am Rev Tuberc.* 1958 Mar;77(3):492-5.

Hata Y, Yamamoto M, Ohni M, Nakajima K, Nakamura Y, Takano T. A placebo-controlled study of the effect of sour milk on blood pressure in hypertensive subjects. *Am J Clin Nutr.* 1996 Nov;64(5):767-71.

Hatakka K, Holma R, El-Nezami H, Suomalainen T, Kuisma M, Saxelin M, Poussa T, Mykkänen H, Korpela R. The influence of *Lactobacillus rhamnosus* LC705 together with Propionibacterium freudenreichii ssp. shermanii JS on potentially carcinogenic bacterial activity in human colon. *Int J Food Microbiol.* 2008 Dec 10;128(2):406-10.

Hattori K, Yamamoto A, Sasai M, Taniuchi S, Kojima T, Kobayashi Y, Iwamoto H, Namba K, Yaeshima T. Effects of administration of bifidobacteria on fecal microflora and clinical symptoms in infants with atopic dermatitis. *Arerugi.* 2003 Jan;52(1):20-30.

He M, Antoine JM, Yang Y, Yang J, Men J, Han H. Influence of live flora on lactose digestion in male adult lactose-malabsorbers after dairy products intake. *Wei Sheng Yan Jiu.* 2004 Sep;33(5):603-5.

He T, Priebe MG, Zhong Y, Huang C, Harmsen HJ, Raangs GC, Antoine JM, Welling GW, Vonk RJ. Effects of yogurt and bifidobacteria supplementation on the colonic microbiota in lactose-intolerant subjects. *J Appl Microbiol.* 2008 Feb;104(2):595-604.

Hickson M, D'Souza AL, Muthu N, Rogers TR, Want S, Rajkumar C, Bulpitt CJ. Use of probiotic Lactobacillus preparation to prevent diarrhoea associated with antibiotics: randomised double blind placebo controlled trial. *BMJ.* 2007 Jul 14;335(7610):80.

Hilton E, Isenberg HD, Alperstein P, France K, Borenstein MT. Ingestion of yogurt containing *Lactobacillus acidophilus* as prophylaxis for *Candida* vaginitis. *Ann Intern Med.* 1992 Mar 1;116(5):353-7.

Hirose Y, Murosaki S, Yamamoto Y, Yoshikai Y, Tsuru T. Daily intake of heat-killed *Lactobacillus plantarum* L-137 augments acquired immunity in healthy adults. *J Nutr.* 2006 Dec;136(12):3069-73.

Hlivak P, Jahnova E, Odraska J, Ferencik M, Ebringer L, Mikes Z. Long-term (56-week) oral administration of probiotic *Enterococcus faecium* M-74 decreases the expression of sICAM-1 and monocyte CD54, and increases that of lymphocyte CD49d in humans. *Bratisl Lek Listy.* 2005;106(4-5):175-81.

Hlivak P, Odraska J, Ferencik M, Ebringer L, Jahnova E, Mikes Z. One-year application of probiotic strain *Enterococcus faecium* M-74 decreases serum cholesterol levels. *Bratisl Lek Listy.* 2005;106(2):67-72.

Hobbs C. *Kombucha Manchurian Tea Mushroom: The Essential Guide.* Santa Cruz, CA: Botanica Press, 1995.

Hobbs C. *Stress & Natural Healing.* Loveland, CO: Interweave Press, 1997.

Hota B, Ellenbogen C, Hayden MK, Aroutcheva A, Rice TW, Weinstein RA. Community-associated methicillin-resistant *Staphylococcus aureus* skin and soft tissue infections at a public hospital: do public housing and incarceration amplify transmission? *Arch Intern Med.* 2007 May 28;167(10):1026-33.

Hoyme UB, Saling E. Efficient prematurity prevention is possible by pH-self measurement and immediate therapy of threatening ascending infection. *Eur J Obstet Gynecol Reprod Biol.* 2004 Aug 10;115(2):148-53.

Hoyos AB. Reduced incidence of necrotizing enterocolitis associated with enteral administration of *Lactobacillus acidophilus* and *Bifidobacterium infantis* to neonates in an intensive care unit. *Int J Infect Dis.* 1999 Summer;3(4):197-202.

Hun L. Bacillus coagulans significantly improved abdominal pain and bloating in patients with IBS. *Postgrad Med.* 2009 Mar;121(2):119-24.

Imase K, Tanaka A, Tokunaga K, Sugano H, Ishida H, Takahashi S. *Lactobacillus reuteri* tablets suppress *Helicobacter pylori* infection—a double-blind randomised placebo-controlled cross-over clinical study. *Kansenshogaku Zasshi.* 2007 Jul;81(4):387-93.

Indrio F, Ladisa G, Mautone A, Montagna O. Effect of a fermented formula on thymus size and stool pH in healthy term infants. *Pediatr Res.* 2007 Jul;62(1):98-100.

Indrio F, Riezzo G, Raimondi F, Bisceglia M, Cavallo L, Francavilla R. The effects of probiotics on feeding tolerance, bowel habits, and gastrointestinal motility in preterm newborns. *J Pediatr.* 2008 Jun;152(6):801-6.

Iovieno A, Lambiase A, Sacchetti M, Stampachiacchiere B, Micera A, Bonini S. Preliminary evidence of the efficacy of probiotic eye-drop treatment in patients with vernal keratoconjunctivitis. *Graefes Arch Clin Exp Ophthalmol.* 2008 Mar;246(3):435-41.

Ishida Y, Nakamura F, Kanzato H, Sawada D, Hirata H, Nishimura A, Kajimoto O, Fujiwara S. Clinical effects of *Lactobacillus acidophilus* strain L-92 on perennial allergic rhinitis: a double-blind, placebo-controlled study. *J Dairy Sci.* 2005 Feb;88(2):527-33.

Ishida Y, Nakamura F, Kanzato H, Sawada D, Yamamoto N, Kagata H, Oh-Ida M, Takeuchi H, Fujiwara S. Effect of milk fermented with *Lactobacillus acidophilus* strain L-92 on symptoms of Japanese cedar pollen allergy: a randomized placebo-controlled trial. *Biosci Biotechnol Biochem.* 2005 Sep;69(9):1652-60.

Ishikawa H, Akedo I, Otani T, Suzuki T, Nakamura T, Takeyama I, Ishiguro S, Miyaoka E, Sobue T, Kakizoe T. Randomized trial of dietary fiber and *Lactobacillus casei* administration for prevention of colorectal tumors. *Int J Cancer.* 2005 Sep 20;116(5):762-7.

Isolauri E, Joensuu J, Suomalainen H, Luomala M, Vesikari T. Improved immunogenicity of oral D x RRV reassortant rotavirus vaccine by *Lactobacillus casei* GG. *Vaccine.* 1995 Feb;13(3):310-2.

Isolauri E, Juntunen M, Rautanen T, Sillanaukee P, Koivula T. A human Lactobacillus strain (*Lactobacillus casei* sp strain GG) promotes recovery from acute diarrhea in children. *Pediatrics.* 1991 Jul;88(1):90-7.

Isolauri E, Kaila M, Mykkänen H, Ling WH, Salminen S. Oral bacteriotherapy for viral gastroenteritis. *Dig Dis Sci.* 1994 Dec;39(12):2595-600.

Ivory K, Chambers SJ, Pin C, Prieto E, Arqués JL, Nicoletti C. Oral delivery of *Lactobacillus casei* Shirota modifies allergen-induced immune responses in allergic rhinitis. *Clin Exp Allergy.* 2008 Aug;38(8):1282-9.

Jacobsen CN, Rosenfeldt Nielsen V, Hayford AE, Moller PL, Michaelsen KF, Paerregaard A, Sandström B, Tvede M, Jakobsen M. Screening of probiotic activities of forty-seven strains of Lactobacillus spp. by in vitro techniques and evaluation of the colonization ability of five selected strains in humans. *Appl Environ Microbiol.* 1999 Nov;65(11):4949-56.

Jain PK, McNaught CE, Anderson AD, MacFie J, Mitchell CJ. Influence of synbiotic containing *Lactobacillus acidophilus* La5, *Bifidobacterium lactis* Bb 12, *Streptococcus thermophilus*, *Lactobacillus bulgaricus* and oligofructose on gut barrier function and sepsis in critically ill patients: a randomised controlled trial. *Clin Nutr.* 2004 Aug;23(4):467-75.

Janelle KC, Barr SI. Nutrient intakes and eating behavior scores of vegetarian and nonvegetarian women. *J Am Diet Assoc.* 1995 Feb;95(2):180-6, 189, quiz 187-8.

Jauhiainen T, Vapaatalo H, Poussa T, Kyrönpalo S, Rasmussen M, Korpela R. *Lactobacillus helveticus* fermented milk lowers blood pressure in hypertensive subjects in 24-h ambulatory blood pressure measurement. *Am J Hypertens.* 2005 Dec;18(12 Pt 1):1600-5.

Jensen B. *Foods that Heal.* Garden City Park, NY: Avery Publ, 1988, 1993.

Jiang T, Mustapha A, Savaiano DA. Improvement of lactose digestion in humans by ingestion of unfermented milk containing *Bifidobacterium longum*. *J Dairy Sci.* 1996 May;79(5):750-7.

Jiménez E, Fernández L, Maldonado A, Martín R, Olivares M, Xaus J, Rodríguez JM. Oral administration of Lactobacillus strains isolated from breast milk as an alternative for the treatment of infectious mastitis during lactation. *Appl Environ Microbiol.* 2008 Aug;74(15):4650-5.

Johansson G, Holmén A, Persson L, Högstedt B, Wassén C, Ottova L, Gustafsson JA. Dietary influence on some proposed risk factors for colon cancer: fecal and urinary mutagenic activity and the activity of some intestinal bacterial enzymes. *Cancer Detect Prev.* 1997;21(3):258-66.

Johansson GK, Ottova L, Gustafsson JA. Shift from a mixed diet to a lactovegetarian diet: influence on some cancer-associated intestinal bacterial enzyme activities. *Nutr Cancer.* 1990;14(3-4):239-46. PubMed PMID: 2128119.

Johansson ML, Nobaek S, Berggren A, Nyman M, Björck I, Ahrné S, Jeppsson B, Molin G. Survival of *Lactobacillus plantarum* DSM 9843 (299v), and effect on the short-chain fatty acid content of faeces after ingestion of a rose-hip drink with fermented oats. *Int J Food Microbiol.* 1998 Jun 30;42(1-2):29-38.

Jones SE, Versalovic J. Probiotic Lactobacillus reuteri biofilms produce antimicrobial and anti-inflammatory factors. *BMC Microbiol.* 2009 Feb 11;9:35.

Kaila M, Isolauri E, Saxelin M, Arvilommi H, Vesikari T. Viable versus inactivated lactobacillus strain GG in acute rotavirus diarrhoea. *Arch Dis Child.* 1995 Jan;72(1):51-3.

Kajander K, Hatakka K, Poussa T, Färkkilä M, Korpela R. A probiotic mixture alleviates symptoms in irritable bowel syndrome patients: a controlled 6-month intervention. *Aliment Pharmacol Ther.* 2005 Sep 1;22(5):387-94.

Kajander K, Korpela R. Clinical studies on alleviating the symptoms of irritable bowel syndrome. *Asia Pac J Clin Nutr.* 2006;15(4):576-80.

Kajander K, Krogius-Kurikka L, Rinttilä T, Karjalainen H, Palva A, Korpela R. Effects of multispecies probiotic supplementation on intestinal microbiota in irritable bowel syndrome. *Aliment Pharmacol Ther.* 2007 Aug 1;26(3):463-73.

Kajander K, Myllyluoma E, Rajilić-Stojanović M, Kyrönpalo S, Rasmussen M, Järvenpää S, Zoetendal EG, de Vos WM, Vapaatalo H, Korpela R. Clinical trial: multispecies probiotic supplementation alleviates the symptoms of irritable bowel syndrome and stabilizes intestinal microbiota. *Aliment Pharmacol Ther.* 2008 Jan 1;27(1):48-57.

Kalliomäki M, Salminen S, Poussa T, Arvilommi H, Isolauri E. Probiotics and prevention of atopic disease: 4-year follow-up of a randomised placebo-controlled trial. *Lancet.* 2003 May 31;361(9372):1869-71.

Kalliomäki M, Salminen S, Poussa T, Isolauri E. Probiotics during the first 7 years of life: a cumulative risk reduction of eczema in a randomized, placebo-controlled trial. *J Allergy Clin Immunol.* 2007 Apr;119(4):1019-21.

Kanazawa H, Nagino M, Kamiya S, Komatsu S, Mayumi T, Takagi K, Asahara T, Nomoto K, Tanaka R, Nimura Y. Synbiotics reduce postoperative infectious complications: a randomized controlled trial in biliary cancer patients undergoing hepatectomy. *Langenbecks Arch Surg.* 2005 Apr;390(2):104-13.

Kankaanpää PE, Yang B, Kallio HP, Isolauri E, Salminen SJ. Influence of probiotic supplemented infant formula on composition of plasma lipids in atopic infants. *J Nutr Biochem.* 2002 Jun;13(6):364-369.

Kano H, Mogami O, Uchida M. Oral administration of milk fermented with Lactobacillus delbrueckii ssp. bulgaricus OLL1073R-1 to DBA/1 mice inhibits secretion of proinflammatory cytokines. *Cytotechnology.* 2002 Nov;40(1-3):67-73.

Kawase M, Hashimoto H, Hosoda M, Morita H, Hosono A. Effect of administration of fermented milk containing whey protein concentrate to rats and healthy men on serum lipids and blood pressure. *J Dairy Sci.* 2000 Feb;83(2):255-63.

Kazansky DB. MHC restriction and allogeneic immune responses. *J Immunotoxicol.* 2008 Oct;5(4):369-84.

Kecskés G, Belágyi T, Oláh A. Early jejunal nutrition with combined pre- and probiotics in acute pancreatitis—prospective, randomized, double-blind investigations. *Magy Seb.* 2003 Feb;56(1):3-8.

Kekkonen RA, Lummela N, Karjalainen H, Latvala S, Tynkkynen S, Jarvenpaa S, Kautiainen H, Julkunen I, Vapaatalo H, Korpela R. Probiotic intervention has strain-specific anti-inflammatory effects in healthy adults. *World J Gastroenterol.* 2008 Apr 7;14(13):2029-36.

Kekkonen RA, Sysi-Aho M, Seppanen-Laakso T, Julkunen I, Vapaatalo H, Oresic M, Korpela R. Effect of probiotic *Lactobacillus rhamnosus* GG intervention on global serum lipidomic profiles in healthy adults. *World J Gastroenterol.* 2008 May 28;14(20):3188-94.

Kekkonen RA, Vasankari TJ, Vuorimaa T, Haahtela T, Julkunen I, Korpela R. The effect of probiotics on respiratory infections and gastrointestinal symptoms during training in marathon runners. *Int J Sport Nutr Exerc Metab.* 2007 Aug;17(4):352-63.

Kiessling G, Schneider J, Jahreis G. Long-term consumption of fermented dairy products over 6 months increases HDL cholesterol. *Eur J Clin Nutr.* 2002 Sep;56(9):843-9.

Kilara A, Shahani KM. The use of immobilized enzymes in the food industry: a review. *CRC Crit Rev Food Sci Nutr.* 1979 Dec;12(2):161-98.

Kim LS, Waters RF, Burkholder PM. Immunological activity of larch arabinogalactan and Echinacea: a preliminary, randomized, double-blind, placebo-controlled trial. *Altern Med Rev.* 2002 Apr;7(2):138-49.

Kim MN, Kim N, Lee SH, Park YS, Hwang JH, Kim JW, Jeong SH, Lee DH, Kim JS, Jung HC, Song IS. The effects of probiotics on PPI-triple therapy for *Helicobacter pylori* eradication. *Helicobacter.* 2008 Aug;13(4):261-8.

Kim YG, Moon JT, Lee KM, Chon NR, Park H. The effects of probiotics on symptoms of irritable bowel syndrome. *Korean J Gastroenterol.* 2006 Jun;47(6):413-9.

Kinross JM, von Roon AC, Holmes E, Darzi A, Nicholson JK. The human gut microbiome: implications for future health care. *Curr Gastroenterol Rep.* 2008 Aug;10(4):396-403.

Kirjavainen PV, Arvola T, Salminen SJ, Isolauri E. Aberrant composition of gut microbiota of allergic infants: a target of bifidobacterial therapy at weaning? *Gut.* 2002 Jul;51(1):51-5.

Kirpich IA, Solovieva NV, Leikhter SN, Shidakova NA, Lebedeva OV, Sidorov PI, Bazhukova TA, Soloviev AG, Barve SS, McClain CJ, Cave M. Probiotics restore bowel flora and improve liver enzymes in human alcohol-induced liver injury: a pilot study. *Alcohol.* 2008 Dec;42(8):675-82.

Kitajima H, Sumida Y, Tanaka R, Yuki N, Takayama H, Fujimura M. Early administration of *Bifidobacterium breve* to preterm infants: randomised controlled trial. *Arch Dis Child Fetal Neonatal Ed.* 1997 Mar;76(2):F101-7.

Klarin B, Johansson ML, Molin G, Larsson A, Jeppsson B. Adhesion of the probiotic bacterium *Lactobacillus plantarum* 299v onto the gut mucosa in critically ill patients: a randomised open trial. *Crit Care.* 2005 Jun;9(3):R285-93.

Klarin B, Molin G, Jeppsson B, Larsson A. Use of the probiotic *Lactobacillus plantarum* 299 to reduce pathogenic bacteria in the oropharynx of intubated patients: a randomised controlled open pilot study. *Crit Care.* 2008;12(6):R136.

Klein A, Friedrich U, Vogelsang H, Jahreis G. *Lactobacillus acidophilus* 74-2 and *Bifidobacterium animalis* subsp *lactis* DGCC 420 modulate unspecific cellular immune response in healthy adults. *Eur J Clin Nutr.* 2008 May;62(5):584-93.

Klein E, Smith D, Laxminarayan R. Trends in Hospitalizations and Deaths in the United States Associated with Infections Caused by Staphylococcus aureus and MRSA, 1999-2004. *Emerging Infectious Diseases. University of Florida Rel.* 2007 Dec 3.

Klein U, Kanellis MJ, Drake D. Effects of four anticaries agents on lesion depth progression in an in vitro caries model. *Pediatr Dent.* 1999 May-Jun;21(3):176-80.

Klima H, Haas O, Roschger P. Photon emission from blood cells and its possible role in immune system regulation. In: Jezowska-Trzebiatowska B. (ed.): *Photon Emission from Biological Systems. Singapore: World Sci.* 1987:153-169.

Klingberg TD, Budde BB. The survival and persistence in the human gastrointestinal tract of five potential probiotic lactobacilli consumed as freeze-dried cultures or as probiotic sausage. *Int J Food Microbiol.* 2006 May 25;109(1-2):157-9.

Kloss J. *Back to Eden.* Twin Oaks, WI: Lotus Press, 1939-1999.

Kollaritsch H, Holst H, Grobara P, Wiedermann G. Prevention of traveler's diarrhea with *Saccharomyces boulardii.* Results of a placebo controlled double-blind study. *Fortschr Med.* 1993 Mar 30;111(9):152-6.

Koop H, Bachem MG. Serum iron, ferritin, and vitamin B12 during prolonged omeprazole therapy. *J Clin Gastroenterol.* 1992;14:288-92.

Korschunov VM, Smeianov VV, Efimov BA, Tarabrina NP, Ivanov AA, Baranov AE. Therapeutic use of an antibiotic-resistant *Bifidobacterium* preparation in men exposed to high-dose gamma-irradiation. *J Med Microbiol.* 1996 Jan;44(1):70-4.

Kotowska M, Albrecht P, Szajewska H. *Saccharomyces boulardii* in the prevention of antibiotic-associated diarrhoea in children: a randomized double-blind placebo-controlled trial. *Aliment Pharmacol Ther.* 2005 Mar 1;21(5):583-90.

Kotzampassi K, Giamarellos-Bourboulis EJ, Voudouris A, Kazamias P, Eleftheriadis E. Benefits of a synbiotic formula (Synbiotic 2000Forte) in critically Ill trauma patients: early results of a randomized controlled trial. *World J Surg.* 2006 Oct;30(10):1848-55.

Krasse P, Carlsson B, Dahl C, Paulsson A, Nilsson A, Sinkiewicz G. Decreased gum bleeding and reduced gingivitis by the probiotic *Lactobacillus reuteri*. *Swed Dent J.* 2006;30(2):55-60.

Kruger K, Kamilli I, Schattenkirchner M. Blastocystis hominis as a rare arthritogenic pathogen. *Z Rheumatol.* 1994 Mar-Apr;53(2):83-5.

Kukkonen K, Nieminen T, Poussa T, Savilahti E, Kuitunen M. Effect of probiotics on vaccine antibody responses in infancy—a randomized placebo-controlled double-blind trial. *Pediatr Allergy Immunol.* 2006 Sep;17(6):416-21.

Kukkonen K, Savilahti E, Haahtela T, Juntunen-Backman K, Korpela R, Poussa T, Tuure T, Kuitunen M. Long-term safety and impact on infection rates of postnatal probiotic and prebiotic (synbiotic) treatment: randomized, double-blind, placebo-controlled trial. *Pediatrics.* 2008 Jul;122(1):8-12.

Kukkonen K, Savilahti E, Haahtela T, Juntunen-Backman K, Korpela R, Poussa T, Tuure T, Kuitunen M. Probiotics and prebiotic galacto-oligosaccharides in the prevention of allergic diseases: a randomized, double-blind, placebo-controlled trial. *J Allergy Clin Immunol.* 2007 Jan;119(1):192-8.

Kurugöl Z, Koturoğlu G. Effects of *Saccharomyces boulardii* in children with acute diarrhoea. *Acta Paediatr.* 2005 Jan;94(1):44-7.

Kuznetsov VF, Iushchuk ND, Iurko LP, Nabokova NIu. Intestinal dysbacteriosis in yersiniosis patients and the possibility of its correction with biopreparations. *Ter Arkh.* 1994;66(11):17-8.

Laitinen K, Isolauri E. Management of food allergy: vitamins, fatty acids or probiotics? *Eur J Gastroenterol Hepatol.* 2005 Dec;17(12):1305-11.

Laitinen K, Poussa T, Isolauri E; Nutrition, Allergy, Mucosal Immunology and Intestinal Microbiota Group. Probiotics and dietary counselling contribute to glucose regulation during and after pregnancy: a randomised controlled trial. *Br J Nutr.* 2009 Jun;101(11):1679-87.

Langhendries JP, Detry J, Van Hees J, Lamboray JM, Darimont J, Mozin MJ, Secretin MC, Senterre J. Effect of a fermented infant formula containing viable bifidobacteria on the fecal flora composition and pH of healthy full-term infants. *J Pediatr Gastroenterol Nutr.* 1995 Aug;21(2):177-81.

Lara-Villoslada F, Sierra S, Boza J, Xaus J, Olivares M. Beneficial effects of consumption of a dairy product containing two probiotic strains, Lactobacillus coryniformis CECT5711 and *Lactobacillus gasseri* CECT5714 in healthy children. *Nutr Hosp.* 2007 Jul-Aug;22(4):496-502.

Leal AL, Eslava-Schmalbach J, Alvarez C, Buitrago G, Méndez M; Grupo para el Control de la Resistencia Bacteriana en Bogotá. Endemic tendencies and bacterial resistance markers in third-level hospitals in Bogotá, Colombia. Rev Salud Publica (Bogota). 2006 May;8 Suppl 1:59-70.

Lee MC, Lin LH, Hung KL, Wu HY. Oral bacterial therapy promotes recovery from acute diarrhea in children. *Acta Paediatr Taiwan.* 2001 Sep-Oct;42(5):301-5.

Lee SJ, Cho SJ, Park EA. Effects of probiotics on enteric flora and feeding tolerance in preterm infants. *Neonatology.* 2007;91(3):174-9.

Lee SJ, Shim YH, Cho SJ, Lee JW. Probiotics prophylaxis in children with persistent primary vesicoureteral reflux. *Pediatr Nephrol.* 2007 Sep;22(9):1315-20.

Lee TH, Hsueh PR, Yeh WC, Wang HP, Wang TH, Lin JT. Low frequency of bacteremia after endoscopic mucosal resection. *Gastrointest Endosc.* 2000 Aug;52(2):223-5.

Lieske JC, Goldfarb DS, De Simone C, Regnier C. Use of a probiotic to decrease enteric hyperoxaluria. *Kidney Int.* 2005 Sep;68(3):1244-9.

Lin HC, Hsu CH, Chen HL, Chung MY, Hsu JF, Lien RI, Tsao LY, Chen CH, Su BH. Oral probiotics prevent necrotizing enterocolitis in very low birth weight preterm infants: a multicenter, randomized, controlled trial. *Pediatrics.* 2008 Oct;122(4):693-700.

Lin HC, Su BH, Chen AC, Lin TW, Tsai CH, Yeh TF, Oh W. Oral probiotics reduce the incidence and severity of necrotizing enterocolitis in very low birth weight infants. *Pediatrics.* 2005 Jan;115(1):1-4.

Lin JS, Chiu YH, Lin NT, Chu CH, Huang KC, Liao KW, Peng KC. Different effects of probiotic species/strains on infections in preschool children: A double-blind, randomized, controlled study. *Vaccine.* 2009 Feb 11;27(7):1073-9.

Lin SY, Ayres JW, Winkler W Jr, Sandine WE. Lactobacillus effects on cholesterol: in vitro and in vivo results. *J Dairy Sci.* 1989 Nov;72(11):2885-99.

Ling WH, Hänninen O. Shifting from a conventional diet to an uncooked vegan diet reversibly alters fecal hydrolytic activities in humans. *J Nutr.* 1992 Apr;122(4):924-30.

Lininger S, Gaby A, Austin S, Brown D, Wright J, Duncan A. *The Natural Pharmacy*. New York: Three Rivers, 1999.

Linsalata M, Russo F, Berloco P, Caruso ML, Matteo GD, Cifone MG, Simone CD, Ierardi E, Di Leo A. The influence of *Lactobacillus brevis* on ornithine decarboxylase activity and polyamine profiles in *Helicobacter pylori*-infected gastric mucosa. *Helicobacter*. 2004 Apr;9(2):165-72.

Lipkind M. Registration of spontaneous photon emission from virus-infected cell cultures: development of experimental system. *Indian J Exp Biol*. 2003 May;41(5):457-72.

Lipski E. *Digestive Wellness*. Los Angeles, CA: Keats, 2000.

Loguercio C, Abbiati R, Rinaldi M, Romano A, Del Vecchio Blanco C, Coltorti M. Long-term effects of *Enterococcus faecium* SF68 versus lactulose in the treatment of patients with cirrhosis and grade 1-2 hepatic encephalopathy. *J Hepatol*. 1995 Jul;23(1):39-46.

Loguercio C, Del Vecchio Blanco C, Coltorti M. Enterococcus lactic acid bacteria strain SF68 and lactulose in hepatic encephalopathy: a controlled study. *J Int Med Res*. 1987 Nov-Dec;15(6):335-43.

Lorea Baroja M, Kirjavainen PV, Hekmat S, Reid G. Anti-inflammatory effects of probiotic yogurt in inflammatory bowel disease patients. *Clin Exp Immunol*. 2007 Sep;149(3):470-9.

Lythcott GI. Anaphylaxis to viomycin. *Am Rev Tuberc*. 1957 Jan;75(1):135-8.

Madden JA, Plummer SF, Tang J, Garaiova I, Plummer NT, Herbison M, Hunter JO, Shimada T, Cheng L, Shirakawa T. Effect of probiotics on preventing disruption of the intestinal microflora following antibiotic therapy: a double-blind, placebo-controlled pilot study. *Int Immunopharmacol*. 2005 Jun;5(6):1091-7.

Mah KW, Chin VI, Wong WS, Lay C, Tannock GW, Shek LP, Aw MM, Chua KY, Wong HB, Panchalingham A, Lee BW. Effect of a milk formula containing probiotics on the fecal microbiota of asian infants at risk of atopic diseases. *Pediatr Res*. 2007 Dec;62(6):674-9.

Majamaa H, Isolauri E, Saxelin M, Vesikari T. Lactic acid bacteria in the treatment of acute rotavirus gastroenteritis. *J Pediatr Gastroenterol Nutr*. 1995 Apr;20(3):333-8.

Manley KJ, Fraenkel MB, Mayall BC, Power DA. Probiotic treatment of vancomycin-resistant enterococci: a randomised controlled trial. *Med J Aust*. 2007 May 7;186(9):454-7.

Manzoni P, Mostert M, Leonessa ML, Priolo C, Farina D, Monetti C, Latino MA, Gomirato G. Oral supplementation with *Lactobacillus casei* subspecies *rhamnosus* prevents enteric colonization by *Candida* species in preterm neonates: a randomized study. *Clin Infect Dis*. 2006 Jun 15;42(12):1735-42.

Marcos A, Wärnberg J, Nova E, Gómez S, Alvarez A, Alvarez R, Mateos JA, Cobo JM. The effect of milk fermented by yogurt cultures plus *Lactobacillus casei* DN-114001 on the immune response of subjects under academic examination stress. *Eur J Nutr*. 2004 Dec;43(6):381-9.

Marteau P, Pochart P, Bouhnik Y, Zidi S, Goderel I, Rambaud JC. Survival of *Lactobacillus acidophilus* and *Bifidobacterium* sp. in the small intestine following ingestion in fermented milk. A rational basis for the use of probiotics in man. *Gastroenterol Clin Biol*. 1992;16(1):25-8.

Martinez RC, Franceschini SA, Patta MC, Quintana SM, Candido RC, Ferreira JC, De Martinis EC, Reid G. Improved treatment of vulvovaginal candidiasis with fluconazole plus probiotic *Lactobacillus rhamnosus* GR-1 and *Lactobacillus reuteri* RC-14. *Lett Appl Microbiol*. 2009 Mar;48(3):269-74.

Martinez RC, Franceschini SA, Patta MC, Quintana SM, Gomes BC, De Martinis EC, Reid G. Improved cure of bacterial vaginosis with single dose of tinidazole (2 g), *Lactobacillus rhamnosus* GR-1, and *Lactobacillus reuteri* RC-14: a randomized, double-blind, placebo-controlled trial. *Can J Microbiol*. 2009 Feb;55(2):133-8.

Martin-Venegas R, Roig-Perez S, Ferrer R, Moreno JJ. Arachidonic acid cascade and epithelial barrier function during Caco-2 cell differentiation. *J Lipid Res*. 2006 Apr;3.

Marushko IuV. The development of a treatment method for streptococcal tonsillitis in children. *Lik Sprava*. 2000 Jan-Feb;(1):79-82.

Masuno T, Kishimoto S, Ogura T, Honma T, Niitani H, Fukuoka M, Ogawa N. A comparative trial of LC9018 plus doxorubicin and doxorubicin alone for the treatment of malignant pleural effusion secondary to lung cancer. *Cancer*. 1991 Oct 1;68(7):1495-500.

Mater DD, Bretigny L, Firmesse O, Flores MJ, Mogenet A, Bresson JL, Corthier G. *Streptococcus thermophilus* and *Lactobacillus delbrueckii* subsp. bulgaricus survive gastrointestinal transit of healthy volunteers consuming yogurt. *FEMS Microbiol Lett*. 2005 Sep 15;250(2):185-7.

Mathur BN, Shahani KM. Use of total whey constituents for human food. *J Dairy Sci*. 1979 Jan;62(1):99-105.

Matsumoto M, Benno Y. Anti-inflammatory metabolite production in the gut from the consumption of probiotic yogurt containing *Bifidobacterium animalis* subsp. *lactis* LKM512. *Biosci Biotechnol Biochem*. 2006 Jun;70(6):1287-92.

Matsumoto M, Benno Y. Consumption of *Bifidobacterium lactis* LKM512 yogurt reduces gut mutagenicity by increasing gut polyamine contents in healthy adult subjects. *Mutat Res*. 2004 Dec 21;568(2):147-53.

Matsuzaki T, Saito M, Usuku K, Nose H, Izumo S, Arimura K, Osame M. A prospective uncontrolled trial of fermented milk drink containing viable *Lactobacillus casei* strain Shirota in the treatment of HTLV-1 associated myelopathy/tropical spastic paraparesis. *J Neurol Sci.* 2005 Oct 15;237(1-2):75-81.

McDougall J, McDougall M. *The McDougal Plan.* Clinton, NJ: New Win, 1983.

McGuire BW, Sia LL, Haynes JD, Kisicki JC, Gutierrez ML, Stokstad EL. Absorption kinetics of orally administered leucovorin calcium. *NCI Monogr.* 1987;(5):47-56.

McGuire BW, Sia LL, Leese PT, Gutierrez ML, Stokstad EL. Pharmacokinetics of leucovorin calcium after intravenous, intramuscular, and oral administration. *Clin Pharm.* 1988 Jan;7(1):52-8.

McNaught CE, Woodcock NP, Anderson AD, MacFie J. A prospective randomised trial of probiotics in critically ill patients. *Clin Nutr.* 2005 Apr;24(2):211-9.

McNaught CE, Woodcock NP, MacFie J, Mitchell CJ. A prospective randomised study of the probiotic *Lactobacillus plantarum* 299V on indices of gut barrier function in elective surgical patients. *Gut.* 2002 Dec;51(6):827-31.

Meyer AL, Elmadfa I, Herbacek I, Micksche M. Probiotic, as well as conventional yogurt, can enhance the stimulated production of proinflammatory cytokines. *J Hum Nutr Diet.* 2007 Dec;20(6):590-8.

Michetti P, Dorta G, Wiesel PH, Brassart D, Verdu E, Herranz M, Felley C, Porta N, Rouvet M, Blum AL, Corthésy-Theulaz I. Effect of whey-based culture supernatant of *Lactobacillus acidophilus* (johnsonii) La1 on *Helicobacter pylori* infection in humans. *Digestion.* 1999;60(3):203-9.

Michielutti F, Bertini M, Presciuttini B, Andreotti G. Clinical assessment of a new oral bacterial treatment for children with acute diarrhea. *Minerva Med.* 1996 Nov;87(11):545-50.

Milgrom P, Ly KA, Roberts MC, Rothen M, Mueller G, Yamaguchi DK. Mutans streptococci dose response to xylitol chewing gum. *J Dent Res.* 2006 Feb;85(2):177-81.

Miller JD, Morin LP, Schwartz WJ, Moore RY. New insights into the mammalian circadian clock. *Sleep.* 1996 Oct;19(8):641-67.

Modern Biology. Austin: Harcourt Brace, 1993.

Mohammad MA, Molloy A, Scott J, Hussein L. Plasma cobalamin and folate and their metabolic markers methylmalonic acid and total homocysteine among Egyptian children before and after nutritional supplementation with the probiotic bacteria *Lactobacillus acidophilus* in yoghurt matrix. *Int J Food Sci Nutr.* 2006 Nov-Dec;57(7-8):470-80.

Mohan R, Koebnick C, Schildt J, Mueller M, Radke M, Blaut M. Effects of *Bifidobacterium lactis* Bb12 supplementation on body weight, fecal pH, acetate, lactate, calprotectin, and IgA in preterm infants. *Pediatr Res.* 2008 Oct;64(4):418-22.

Mohan R, Koebnick C, Schildt J, Schmidt S, Mueller M, Possner M, Radke M, Blaut M. Effects of *Bifidobacterium lactis* Bb12 supplementation on intestinal microbiota of preterm infants: a double-blind, placebo-controlled, randomized study. *J Clin Microbiol.* 2006 Nov;44(11):4025-31.

Morimoto K, Takeshita T, Nanno M, Tokudome S, Nakayama K. Modulation of natural killer cell activity by supplementation of fermented milk containing *Lactobacillus casei* in habitual smokers. *Prev Med.* 2005 May;40(5):589-94.

Moss M. E. Coli Path Shows Flaws in Ground Beef Inspection. *NY Times* 2009 Oct 3.

Mozafar A. Is there vitamin B12 in plants or not? A plant nutritionist's view. *Veg Nutr.* 1997;1/2:50-52.

Mullié C, Yazourh A, Thibault H, Odou MF, Singer E, Kalach N, Kremp O, Romond MB. Increased poliovirus-specific intestinal antibody response coincides with promotion of *Bifidobacterium longum-infantis* and *Bifidobacterium breve* in infants: a randomized, double-blind, placebo-controlled trial. *Pediatr Res.* 2004 Nov;56(5):791-5.

Murray M and Pizzorno J. *Encyclopedia of Natural Medicine.* 2nd Edition. Roseville, CA: Prima Publishing, 1998.

Mustapha A, Jiang T, Savaiano DA. Improvement of lactose digestion by humans following ingestion of unfermented acidophilus milk: influence of bile sensitivity, lactose transport, and acid tolerance of *Lactobacillus acidophilus.* J Dairy Sci. 1997 Aug;80(8):1537-45.

Myllyluoma E, Ahonen AM, Korpela R, Vapaatalo H, Kankuri E. Effects of multispecies probiotic combination on helicobacter pylori infection in vitro. *Clin Vaccine Immunol.* 2008 Sep;15(9):1472-82.

Naito S, Koga H, Yamaguchi A, Fujimoto N, Hasui Y, Kuramoto H, Iguchi A, Kinukawa N; Kyushu University Urological Oncology Group. Prevention of recurrence with epirubicin and *Lactobacillus casei* after transurethral resection of bladder cancer. *J Urol.* 2008 Feb;179(2):485-90.

Naruszewicz M, Johansson ML, Zapolska-Downar D, Bukowska H. Effect of *Lactobacillus plantarum* 299v on cardiovascular disease risk factors in smokers. *Am J Clin Nutr.* 2002 Dec;76(6):1249-55.

Narva M, Nevala R, Poussa T, Korpela R. The effect of *Lactobacillus helveticus* fermented milk on acute changes in calcium metabolism in postmenopausal women. *Eur J Nutr.* 2004 Apr;43(2):61-8.

REFERENCES AND BIBLIOGRAPHY

Näse L, Hatakka K, Savilahti E, Saxelin M, Pönkä A, Poussa T, Korpela R, Meurman JH. Effect of long-term consumption of a probiotic bacterium, *Lactobacillus rhamnosus* GG, in milk on dental caries and caries risk in children. *Caries Res.* 2001 Nov-Dec;35(6):412-20.

Niedzielin K, Kordecki H, Birkenfeld B. A controlled, double-blind, randomized study on the efficacy of *Lactobacillus plantarum* 299V in patients with irritable bowel syndrome. *Eur J Gastroenterol Hepatol.* 2001 Oct;13(10):1143-7.

Nielsen OH, Jorgensen S, Pedersen K, Justesen T. Microbiological evaluation of jejunal aspirates and faecal samples after oral administration of bifidobacteria and lactic acid bacteria. *J Appl Bacteriol.* 1994 May;76(5):469-74.

Nilson KM, Vakil JR, Shahani KM. B-complex vitamin content of cheddar cheese. *J Nutr.* 1965 Aug;86:362-8.

Nobaek S, Johansson ML, Molin G, Ahrné S, Jeppsson B. Alteration of intestinal microflora is associated with reduction in abdominal bloating and pain in patients with irritable bowel syndrome. *Am J Gastroenterol.* 2000 May;95(5):1231-8.

Nopchinda S, Varavithya W, Phuapradit P, Sangchai R, Suthutvoravut U, Chantraruksa V, Haschke F. Effect of bifidobacterium Bb12 with or without *Streptococcus thermophilus* supplemented formula on nutritional status. *J Med Assoc Thai.* 2002 Nov;85 Suppl 4:S1225-31.

Nova E, Toro O, Varela P, López-Vidriero I, Morandé G, Marcos A. Effects of a nutritional intervention with yogurt on lymphocyte subsets and cytokine production capacity in anorexia nervosa patients. *Eur J Nutr.* 2006 Jun;45(4):225-33.

O'Brien SJ, Shannon JE, Gail MH. A molecular approach to the identification and individualization of human and animal cells in culture: isozyme and allozyme genetic signatures. *In Vitro.* 1980 Feb;16(2):119-35.

Odamaki T, Xiao JZ, Iwabuchi N, Sakamoto M, Takahashi N, Kondo S, Miyaji K, Iwatsuki K, Togashi H, Enomoto T, Benno Y. Influence of *Bifidobacterium longum* BB536 intake on faecal microbiota in individuals with Japanese cedar pollinosis during the pollen season. *J Med Microbiol.* 2007 Oct;56(Pt 10):1301-8.

Odamaki T, Xiao JZ, Iwabuchi N, Sakamoto M, Takahashi N, Kondo S, Iwatsuki K, Kokubo S, Togashi H, Enomoto T, Benno Y. Fluctuation of fecal microbiota in individuals with Japanese cedar pollinosis during the pollen season and influence of probiotic intake. *J Investig Allergol Clin Immunol.* 2007;17(2):92-100.

Ogawa T, Hashikawa S, Asai Y, Sakamoto H, Yasuda K, Makimura Y. A new synbiotic, *Lactobacillus casei* subsp. casei together with dextran, reduces murine and human allergic reaction. *FEMS Immunol Med Microbiol.* 2006 Apr;46(3):400-9.

Ohashi Y, Nakai S, Tsukamoto T, Masumori N, Akaza H, Miyanaga N, Kitamura T, Kawabe K, Kotake T, Kuroda M, Naito S, Koga H, Saito Y, Nomata K, Kitagawa M, Aso Y. Habitual intake of lactic acid bacteria and risk reduction of bladder cancer. *Urol Int.* 2002;68(4):273-80.

Okamura T, Maehara Y, Sugimachi K. Phase II clinical study of LC9018 on carcinomatous peritonitis of gastric cancer. Subgroup for Carcinomatous Peritonitis, Cooperative, Study Group of LC9018. *Gan To Kagaku Ryoho.* 1989 Jun;16(6):2257-62.

Okawa T, Niibe H, Arai T, Sekiba K, Noda K, Takeuchi S, Hashimoto S, Ogawa N. Effect of LC9018 combined with radiation therapy on carcinoma of the uterine cervix. A phase III, multicenter, randomized, controlled study. *Cancer.* 1993 Sep 15;72(6):1949-54.

Oláh A, Belágyi T, Issekutz A, Gamal ME, Bengmark S. Randomized clinical trial of specific lactobacillus and fibre supplement to early enteral nutrition in patients with acute pancreatitis. *Br J Surg.* 2002 Sep;89(9):1103-7.

Oleĭnichenko EV, Mitrokhin SD, Nonikov VE, Minaev VI. Effectiveness of acipole in prevention of enteric dysbacteriosis due to antibacterial therapy. *Antibiot Khimioter.* 1999;44(1):23-5.

Olivares M, Díaz-Ropero MA, Gómez N, Lara-Villoslada F, Sierra S, Maldonado JA, Martín R, López-Huertas E, Rodríguez JM, Xaus J. Oral administration of two probiotic strains, *Lactobacillus gasseri* CECT5714 and Lactobacillus coryniformis CECT5711, enhances the intestinal function of healthy adults. *Int J Food Microbiol.* 2006 Mar 15;107(2):104-11.

Olivares M, Paz Díaz-Ropero M, Gómez N, Sierra S, Lara-Villoslada F, Martín R, Miguel Rodríguez J, Xaus J. Dietary deprivation of fermented foods causes a fall in innate immune response. Lactic acid bacteria can counteract the immunological effect of this deprivation. *J Dairy Res.* 2006 Nov;73(4):492-8.

O'Mahony L, McCarthy J, Kelly P, Hurley G, Luo F, Chen K, O'Sullivan GC, Kiely B, Collins JK, Shanahan F, Quigley EM. Lactobacillus and bifidobacterium in irritable bowel syndrome: symptom responses and relationship to cytokine profiles. *Gastroenterology.* 2005 Mar;128(3):541-51.

Onwulata CI, Rao DR, Vankineni P. Relative efficiency of yogurt, sweet acidophilus milk, hydrolyzed-lactose milk, and a commercial lactase tablet in alleviating lactose maldigestion. *Am J Clin Nutr.* 1989 Jun;49(6):1233-7.

Oozeer R, Leplingard A, Mater DD, Mogenet A, Michelin R, Seksek I, Marteau P, Doré J, Bresson JL, Corthier G. Survival of *Lactobacillus casei* in the human digestive tract after consumption of fermented milk. *Appl Environ Microbiol.* 2006 Aug;72(8):5615-7.

Ortiz-Andrellucchi A, Sánchez-Villegas A, Rodríguez-Gallego C, Lemes A, Molero T, Soria A, Peña-Quintana L, Santana M, Ramírez O, García J, Cabrera F, Cobo J, Serra-Majem L. Immunomodulatory effects of the intake of fermented milk with *Lactobacillus casei* DN114001 in lactating mothers and their children. *Br J Nutr.* 2008 Oct;100(4):834-45.

Ouwehand AC, Bergsma N, Parhiala R, Lahtinen S, Gueimonde M, Finne-Soveri H, Strandberg T, Pitkälä K, Salminen S. *Bifidobacterium* microbiota and parameters of immune function in elderly subjects. *FEMS Immunol Med Microbiol.* 2008 Jun;53(1):18-25.

Ouwehand AC, Tiihonen K, Saarinen M, Putaala H, Rautonen N. Influence of a combination of *Lactobacillus acidophilus* NCFM and lactitol on healthy elderly: intestinal and immune parameters. *Br J Nutr.* 2009 Feb;101(3):367-75.

Ouwehand AC. Antiallergic effects of probiotics. *J Nutr.* 2007 Mar;137(3 Suppl 2):794S-7S.

Ozkan TB, Sahin E, Erdemir G, Budak F. Effect of *Saccharomyces boulardii* in children with acute gastroenteritis and its relationship to the immune response. *J Int Med Res.* 2007 Mar-Apr;35(2):201-12.

Paineau D, Carcano D, Leyer G, Darquy S, Alyanakian MA, Simoneau G, Bergmann JF, Brassart D, Bornet F, Ouwehand AC. Effects of seven potential probiotic strains on specific immune responses in healthy adults: a double-blind, randomized, controlled trial. *FEMS Immunol Med Microbiol.* 2008 Jun;53(1):107-13.

Panigrahi P, Parida S, Pradhan L, Mohapatra SS, Misra PR, Johnson JA, Chaudhry R, Taylor S, Hansen NI, Gewolb IH. Long-term colonization of a *Lactobacillus plantarum* synbiotic preparation in the neonatal gut. *J Pediatr Gastroenterol Nutr.* 2008 Jul;47(1):45-53.

Parra D, De Morentin BM, Cobo JM, Mateos A, Martinez JA. Monocyte function in healthy middle-aged people receiving fermented milk containing *Lactobacillus casei*. *J Nutr Health Aging.* 2004;8(4):208-11.

Parra MD, Martínez de Morentin BE, Cobo JM, Mateos A, Martínez JA. Daily ingestion of fermented milk containing *Lactobacillus casei* DN114001 improves innate-defense capacity in healthy middle-aged people. *J Physiol Biochem.* 2004 Jun;60(2):85-91.

Passeron T, Lacour JP, Fontas E, Ortonne JP. Prebiotics and synbiotics: two promising approaches for the treatment of atopic dermatitis in children above 2 years. *Allergy.* 2006 Apr;61(4):431-7.

Patterson DB. Anaphylactic shock from chloromycetin. Northwest Med. 1950 May;49(5):352-3.Agarwal KN, Bhasin SK. Feasibility studies to control acute diarrhoea in children by feeding fermented milk preparations Actimel and Indian Dahi. *Eur J Clin Nutr.* 2002 Dec;56 Suppl 4:S56-9.

Pedone CA, Arnaud CC, Postaire ER, Bouley CF, Reinert P. Multicentric study of the effect of milk fermented by *Lactobacillus casei* on the incidence of diarrhoea. *Int J Clin Pract.* 2000 Nov;54(9):568-71.

Pedone CA, Bernabeu AO, Postaire ER, Bouley CF, Reinert P. The effect of supplementation with milk fermented by *Lactobacillus casei* (strain DN-114 001) on acute diarrhoea in children attending day care centres. *Int J Clin Pract.* 1999 Apr-May;53(3):179-84.

Pedrosa MC, Golner BB, Goldin BR, Barakat S, Dallal GE, Russell RM. Survival of yogurt-containing organisms and *Lactobacillus gasseri* (ADH) and their effect on bacterial enzyme activity in the gastrointestinal tract of healthy and hypochlorhydric elderly subjects. *Am J Clin Nutr.* 1995 Feb;61(2):353-9.

Peral MC, Martinez MA, Valdez JC. Bacteriotherapy with *Lactobacillus plantarum* in burns. *Int Wound J.* 2009 Feb;6(1):73-81.

Persson R, Orbaek P, Kecklund G, Akerstedt T. Impact of an 84-hour workweek on biomarkers for stress, metabolic processes and diurnal rhythm. *Scand J Work Environ Health.* 2006 Oct;32(5):349-58.

Pessi T, Sütas Y, Hurme M, Isolauri E. Interleukin-10 generation in atopic children following oral *Lactobacillus rhamnosus* GG. *Clin Exp Allergy.* 2000 Dec;30(12):1804-8.

Petricevic L, Unger FM, Viernstein H, Kiss H. Randomized, double-blind, placebo-controlled study of oral lactobacilli to improve the vaginal flora of postmenopausal women. *Eur J Obstet Gynecol Reprod Biol.* 2008 Nov;141(1):54-7.

Petricevic L, Witt A. The role of *Lactobacillus casei* rhamnosus Lcr35 in restoring the normal vaginal flora after antibiotic treatment of bacterial vaginosis. *BJOG.* 2008 Oct;115(11):1369-74.

Petrunov B, Marinova S, Markova R, Nenkov P, Nikolaeva S, Nikolova M, Taskov H, Cvetanov J. Cellular and humoral systemic and mucosal immune responses stimulated in volunteers by an oral polybacterial immunomodulator "Dentavax". *Int Immunopharmacol.* 2006 Jul;6(7):1181-93.

Petti S, Tarsitani G, D'Arca AS. A randomized clinical trial of the effect of yoghurt on the human salivary microflora. *Arch Oral Biol.* 2001 Aug;46(8):705-12.

Phuapradit P, Varavithya W, Vathanophas K, Sangchai R, Podhipak A, Suthutvoravut U, Nopchinda S, Chantraruksa V, Haschke F. Reduction of rotavirus infection in children receiving bifidobacteria-supplemented formula. *J Med Assoc Thai.* 1999 Nov;82 Suppl 1:S43-8.

Piirainen L, Haahtela S, Helin T, Korpela R, Haahtela T, Vaarala O. Effect of *Lactobacillus rhamnosus* GG on rBet v1 and rMal d1 specific IgA in the saliva of patients with birch pollen allergy. *Ann Allergy Asthma Immunol.* 2008 Apr;100(4):338-42.

Pitkala KH, Strandberg TE, Finne Soveri UH, Ouwehand AC, Poussa T, Salminen S. Fermented cereal with specific bifidobacteria normalizes bowel movements in elderly nursing home residents. A randomized, controlled trial. *J Nutr Health Aging.* 2007 Jul-Aug;11(4):305-11.

Plein K, Hotz J. Therapeutic effects of *Saccharomyces boulardii* on mild residual symptoms in a stable phase of Crohn's disease with special respect to chronic diarrhea—a pilot study. *Z Gastroenterol.* 1993 Feb;31(2):129-34.

Pohjavuori E, Viljanen M, Korpela R, Kuitunen M, Tiittanen M, Vaarala O, Savilahti E. Lactobacillus GG effect in increasing IFN-gamma production in infants with cow's milk allergy. *J Allergy Clin Immunol.* 2004 Jul;114(1):131-6.

Pregliasco F, Anselmi G, Fonte L, Giussani F, Schieppati S, Soletti L. A new chance of preventing winter diseases by the administration of synbiotic formulations. *J Clin Gastroenterol.* 2008 Sep;42 Suppl 3 Pt 2:S224-33.

Prescott SL, Wickens K, Westcott L, Jung W, Currie H, Black PN, Stanley TV, Mitchell EA, Fitzharris P, Siebers R, Wu L, Crane J; Probiotic Study Group. Supplementation with *Lactobacillus rhamnosus* or *Bifidobacterium lactis* probiotics in pregnancy increases cord blood interferon-gamma and breast milk transforming growth factor-beta and immunoglobin A detection. *Clin Exp Allergy.* 2008 Oct;38(10):1606-14.

Qin HL, Zheng JJ, Tong DN, Chen WX, Fan XB, Hang XM, Jiang YQ. Effect of *Lactobacillus plantarum* enteral feeding on the gut permeability and septic complications in the patients with acute pancreatitis. *Eur J Clin Nutr.* 2008 Jul;62(7):923-30.

Rafter J, Bennett M, Caderni G, Clune Y, Hughes R, Karlsson PC, Klinder A, O'Riordan M, O'Sullivan GC, Pool-Zobel B, Rechkemmer G, Roller M, Rowland I, Salvadori M, Thijs H, Van Loo J, Watzl B, Collins JK. Dietary synbiotics reduce cancer risk factors in polypectomized and colon cancer patients. *Am J Clin Nutr.* 2007 Feb;85(2):488-96.

Randal Bollinger R, Barbas AS, Bush EL, Lin SS, Parker W. Biofilms in the large bowel suggest an apparent function of the human vermiform appendix. *J Theor Biol.* 2007 Dec 21;249(4):826-31.

Rangavajhyala N, Shahani KM, Sridevi G, Srikumaran S. Nonlipopolysaccharide component(s) of Lactobacillus acidophilus stimulate(s) the production of interleukin-1 alpha and tumor necrosis factor-alpha by murine macrophages. *Nutr Cancer.* 1997;28(2):130-4.

Rautava S, Salminen S, Isolauri E. Specific probiotics in reducing the risk of acute infections in infancy—a randomised, double-blind, placebo-controlled study. *Br J Nutr.* 2009 Jun;101(11):1722-6.

Rayes N, Seehofer D, Hansen S, Boucsein K, Müller AR, Serke S, Bengmark S, Neuhaus P. Early enteral supply of lactobacillus and fiber versus selective bowel decontamination: a controlled trial in liver transplant recipients. *Transplantation.* 2002 Jul 15;74(1):123-7.

Rayes N, Seehofer D, Müller AR, Hansen S, Bengmark S, Neuhaus P. Influence of probiotics and fibre on the incidence of bacterial infections following major abdominal surgery - results of a prospective trial. *Z Gastroenterol.* 2002 Oct;40(10):869-76.

Raza S, Graham SM, Allen SJ, Sultana S, Cuevas L, Hart CA, Kaila M, Isolauri E, Saxelin M, Arvilommi H, et al. Lactobacillus GG in acute diarrhea. *Indian Pediatr.* 1995 Oct;32(10):1140-2.

Raza S, Graham SM, Allen SJ, Sultana S, Cuevas L, Hart CA. Lactobacillus GG promotes recovery from acute nonbloody diarrhea in Pakistan. Pediatr Infect Dis J. 1995 Feb;14(2):107-11.

Reddy KP, Shahani KM, Kulkarni SM. B-complex vitamins in cultured and acidified yogurt. *J Dairy Sci.* 1976 Feb;59(2):191-5.

Reger D, Goode S, Mercer E. *Chemistry: Principles & Practice.* Fort Worth, TX: Harcourt Brace, 1993.

Regis E. *Virus Ground Zero.* New York: Pocket, 1996.

Reid G, Beuerman D, Heinemann C, Bruce AW. Probiotic Lactobacillus dose required to restore and maintain a normal vaginal flora. *FEMS Immunol Med Microbiol.* 2001 Dec;32(1):37-41.

Reid G, Burton J, Hammond JA, Bruce AW. Nucleic acid-based diagnosis of bacterial vaginosis and improved management using probiotic lactobacilli. *J Med Food.* 2004 Summer;7(2):223-8.

Reid G, Charbonneau D, Erb J, Kochanowski B, Beuerman D, Poehner R, Bruce AW. Oral use of *Lactobacillus rhamnosus* GR-1 and L. fermentum RC-14 significantly alters vaginal flora: randomized, placebo-controlled trial in 64 healthy women. *FEMS Immunol Med Microbiol.* 2003 Mar 20;35(2):131-4.

Renvert S, Lindahl C, Renvert H, Persson GR. Clinical and microbiological analysis of subjects treated with Brånemark or AstraTech implants: a 7-year follow-up study. *Clin Oral Implants Res.* 2008 Apr;19(4):342-7.

Riccia DN, Bizzini F, Perilli MG, Polimeni A, Trinchieri V, Amicosante G, Cifone MG. Anti-inflammatory effects of *Lactobacillus brevis* (CD2) on periodontal disease. *Oral Dis.* 2007 Jul;13(4):376-85.

Rinne M, Kalliomaki M, Arvilommi H, Salminen S, Isolauri E. Effect of probiotics and breastfeeding on the bifidobacterium and lactobacillus/enterococcus microbiota and humoral immune responses. *J Pediatr.* 2005 Aug;147(2):186-91.

Rinne M, Kalliomäki M, Salminen S, Isolauri E. Probiotic intervention in the first months of life: short-term effects on gastrointestinal symptoms and long-term effects on gut microbiota. *J Pediatr Gastroenterol Nutr.* 2006 Aug;43(2):200-5.

Río ME, Zago Beatriz L, Garcia H, Winter L. The nutritional status change the effectiveness of a dietary supplement of lactic bacteria on the emerging of respiratory tract diseases in children. *Arch Latinoam Nutr.* 2002 Mar;52(1):29-34.

Río ME, Zago LB, Garcia H, Winter L. Influence of nutritional status on the effectiveness of a dietary supplement of live lactobacillus to prevent and cure diarrhoea in children. *Arch Latinoam Nutr.* 2004 Sep;54(3):287-92.

Roessler A, Friedrich U, Vogelsang H, Bauer A, Kaatz M, Hipler UC, Schmidt I, Jahreis G. The immune system in healthy adults and patients with atopic dermatitis seems to be affected differently by a probiotic intervention. *Clin Exp Allergy.* 2008 Jan;38(1):93-102.

Roller M, Clune Y, Collins K, Rechkemmer G, Watzl B. Consumption of prebiotic inulin enriched with oligofructose in combination with the probiotics *Lactobacillus rhamnosus* and *Bifidobacterium lactis* has minor effects on selected immune parameters in polypectomised and colon cancer patients. *Br J Nutr.* 2007 Apr;97(4):676-84.

Rosander A, Connolly E, Roos S. Removal of antibiotic resistance gene-carrying plasmids from *Lactobacillus reuteri* ATCC 55730 and characterization of the resulting daughter strain, *L. reuteri* DSM 17938. *Appl Environ Microbiol.* 2008 Oct;74(19):6032-40.

Rosenfeldt V, Benfeldt E, Valerius NH, Paerregaard A, Michaelsen KF. Effect of probiotics on gastrointestinal symptoms and small intestinal permeability in children with atopic dermatitis. *J Pediatr.* 2004 Nov;145(5):612-6.

Rousseaux C, Thuru X, Gelot A, Barnich N, Neut C, Dubuquoy L, Dubuquoy C, Merour E, Geboes K, Chamaillard M, Ouwehand A, Leyer G, Carcano D, Colombel JF, Ardid D, Desreumaux P. Lactobacillus acidophilus modulates intestinal pain and induces opioid and cannabinoid receptors. *Nat Med.* 2007 Jan;13(1):35-7

Saavedra JM, Abi-Hanna A, Moore N, Yolken RH. Long-term consumption of infant formulas containing live probiotic bacteria: tolerance and safety. *Am J Clin Nutr.* 2004 Feb;79(2):261-7.

Saavedra JM, Bauman NA, Oung I, Perman JA, Yolken RH. Feeding of *Bifidobacterium bifidum* and *Streptococcus thermophilus* to infants in hospital for prevention of diarrhoea and shedding of rotavirus. *Lancet.* 1994 Oct 15;344(8929):1046-9.

Saggioro A. Probiotics in the treatment of irritable bowel syndrome. *J Clin Gastroenterol.* 2004 Jul;38(6 Suppl):S104-6.

Sahagún-Flores JE, López-Peña LS, de la Cruz-Ramírez Jaimes J, García-Bravo MS, Peregrina-Gómez R, de Alba-García JE. Eradication of *Helicobacter pylori*: triple treatment scheme plus Lactobacillus vs. triple treatment alone. *Cir Cir.* 2007 Sep-Oct;75(5):333-6.

Salazar-Lindo E, Figueroa-Quintanilla D, Caciano MI, Reto-Valiente V, Chauviere G, Colin P; Lacteol Study Group. Effectiveness and safety of Lactobacillus LB in the treatment of mild acute diarrhea in children. *J Pediatr Gastroenterol Nutr.* 2007 May;44(5):571-6.

Salazar-Lindo E, Miranda-Langschwager P, Campos-Sanchez M, Chea-Woo E, Sack RB. *Lactobacillus casei* strain GG in the treatment of infants with acute watery diarrhea: a randomized, double-blind, placebo controlled clinical trial [ISRCTN67363048]. *BMC Pediatr.* 2004 Sep 2;4:18.

Salminen E, Elomaa I, Minkkinen J, Vapaatalo H, Salminen S. Preservation of intestinal integrity during radiotherapy using live *Lactobacillus acidophilus* cultures. *Clin Radiol.* 1988 Jul;39(4):435-7.

Samanta M, Sarkar M, Ghosh P, Ghosh J, Sinha M, Chatterjee S. Prophylactic probiotics for prevention of necrotizing enterocolitis in very low birth weight newborns. *J Trop Pediatr.* 2009 Apr;55(2):128-31.

Saran S, Gopalan S, Krishna TP. Use of fermented foods to combat stunting and failure to thrive. *Nutrition.* 2002 May;18(5):393-6.

Savino F, Pelle E, Palumeri E, Oggero R, Miniero R. *Lactobacillus reuteri* (American Type Culture Collection Strain 55730) versus simethicone in the treatment of infantile colic: a prospective randomized study. Pediatrics. 2007 Jan;119(1):e124-30.

Schaafsma G, Meuling WJ, van Dokkum W, Bouley C. Effects of a milk product, fermented by *Lactobacillus acidophilus* and with fructo-oligosaccharides added, on blood lipids in male volunteers. *Eur J Clin Nutr.* 1998 Jun;52(6):436-40.

REFERENCES AND BIBLIOGRAPHY

Schiffrin EJ, Brassart D, Servin AL, Rochat F, Donnet-Hughes A. Immune modulation of blood leukocytes in humans by lactic acid bacteria: criteria for strain selection. *Am J Clin Nutr.* 1997 Aug;66(2):515S-520S.

Scholz-Ahrens KE, Ade P, Marten B, Weber P, Timm W, Açil Y, Glüer CC, Schrezenmeir J. Prebiotics, probiotics, and synbiotics affect mineral absorption, bone mineral content, and bone structure. *J Nutr.* 2007 Mar;137(3 Suppl 2):838S-46S.

Schulman G. A nexus of progression of chronic kidney disease: charcoal, tryptophan and profibrotic cytokines. *Blood Purif.* 2006;24(1):143-8.

Schumacher P. *Biophysical Therapy Of Allergies.* Stuttgart: Thieme, 2005.

Sekine K, Toida T, Saito M, Kuboyama M, Kawashima T, Hashimoto Y. A new morphologically characterized cell wall preparation (whole peptidoglycan) from *Bifidobacterium* infantis with a higher efficacy on the regression of an established tumor in mice. *Cancer Res.* 1985 Mar;45(3):1300-7.

Seppo L, Jauhiainen T, Poussa T, Korpela R. A fermented milk high in bioactive peptides has a blood pressure-lowering effect in hypertensive subjects. *Am J Clin Nutr.* 2003 Feb;77(2):326-30.

Shahani KM, Ayebo AD. Role of dietary lactobacilli in gastrointestinal microecology. *Am J Clin Nutr.* 1980 Nov;33(11 Suppl):2448-57.

Shahani KM, Chandan RC. Nutritional and healthful aspects of cultured and culture-containing dairy foods. *J Dairy Sci.* 1979 Oct;62(10):1685-94.

Shahani KM, Friend BA. Properties of and prospects for cultured dairy foods. *Soc Appl Bacteriol Symp Ser.* 1983;11:257-69.

Shahani KM, Herper WJ, Jensen RG, Parry RM Jr, Zittle CA. Enzymes in bovine milk: a review. *J Dairy Sci.* 1973 May;56(5):531-43.

Shahani KM, Kwan AJ, Friend BA. Role and significance of enzymes in human milk. *Am J Clin Nutr.* 1980 Aug;33(8):1861-8.

Shahani KM, Meshbesher BF, Mangalampalli V. *Cultivate Health From Within.* Vital Health Publ: Danbury, CT, 2005.

Shalev E, Battino S, Weiner E, Colodner R, Keness Y. Ingestion of yogurt containing *Lactobacillus acidophilus* compared with pasteurized yogurt as prophylaxis for recurrent *Candida* vaginitis and bacterial vaginosis. *Arch Fam Med.* 1996 Nov-Dec;5(10):593-6.

Shamir R, Makhoul IR, Etzioni A, Shehadeh N. Evaluation of a diet containing probiotics and zinc for the treatment of mild diarrheal illness in children younger than one year of age. *J Am Coll Nutr.* 2005 Oct;24(5):370-5.

Sharma P, Sharma BC, Puri V, Sarin SK. An open-label randomized controlled trial of lactulose and probiotics in the treatment of minimal hepatic encephalopathy. *Eur J Gastroent Hepatol.* 2008 Jun;20(6):506-11.

Sheih YH, Chiang BL, Wang LH, Liao CK, Gill HS. Systemic immunity-enhancing effects in healthy subjects following dietary consumption of the lactic acid bacterium *Lactobacillus rhamnosus* HN001. *J Am Coll Nutr.* 2001 Apr;20(2 Suppl):149-56.

Shimauchi H, Mayanagi G, Nakaya S, Minamibuchi M, Ito Y, Yamaki K, Hirata H. Improvement of periodontal condition by probiotics with *Lactobacillus salivarius* WB21: a randomized, double-blind, placebo-controlled study. *J Clin Periodontol.* 2008 Oct;35(10):897-905.

Shimizu K, Ogura H, Goto M, Asahara T, Nomoto K, Morotomi M, Matsushima A, Tasaki O, Fujita K, Hosotsubo H, Kuwagata Y, Tanaka H, Shimazu T, Sugimoto H. Synbiotics decrease the incidence of septic complications in patients with severe SIRS: a preliminary report. *Dig Dis Sci.* 2009 May;54(5):1071-8.

Shoaf K, Mulvey GL, Armstrong GD, Hutkins RW. Prebiotic galactooligosaccharides reduce adherence of enteropathogenic *Escherichia coli* to tissue culture cells. *Infect Immun.* 2006 Dec;74(12):6920-8.

Shornikova AV, Casas IA, Isolauri E, Mykkänen H, Vesikari T. *Lactobacillus reuteri* as a therapeutic agent in acute diarrhea in young children. *J Pediatr Gastroenterol Nutr.* 1997 Apr;24(4):399-404.

Shornikova AV, Casas IA, Mykkänen H, Salo E, Vesikari T. Bacteriotherapy with *Lactobacillus reuteri* in rotavirus gastroenteritis. *Pediatr Infect Dis J.* 1997 Dec;16(12):1103-7.

Silva MR, Dias G, Ferreira CL, Franceschini SC, Costa NM. Growth of preschool children was improved when fed an iron-fortified fermented milk beverage supplemented with *Lactobacillus acidophilus. Nutr Res.* 2008 Apr;28(4):226-32.

Simakachorn N, Pichaipat V, Rithipornpaisarn P, Kongkaew C, Tongpradit P, Varavithya W. Clinical evaluation of the addition of lyophilized, heat-killed *Lactobacillus acidophilus* LB to oral rehydration therapy in the treatment of acute diarrhea in children. *J Pediatr Gastroenterol Nutr.* 2000 Jan;30(1):68-72.

Simenhoff ML, Dunn SR, Zollner GP, Fitzpatrick ME, Emery SM, Sandine WE, Ayres JW. Biomodulation of the toxic and nutritional effects of small bowel bacterial overgrowth in end-stage kidney disease using freeze-dried *Lactobacillus acidophilus. Miner Electrolyte Metab.* 1996;22(1-3):92-6.

PROBIOTICS — PROTECTION AGAINST INFECTION

Sinn DH, Song JH, Kim HJ, Lee JH, Son HJ, Chang DK, Kim YH, Kim JJ, Rhee JC, Rhee PL. Therapeutic effect of *Lactobacillus acidophilus*-SDC 2012, 2013 in patients with irritable bowel syndrome. *Dig Dis Sci.* 2008 Oct;53(10):2714-8.

Sistek D, Kelly R, Wickens K, Stanley T, Fitzharris P, Crane J. Is the effect of probiotics on atopic dermatitis confined to food sensitized children? *Clin Exp Allergy.* 2006 May;36(5):629-33.

Skovbjerg S, Roos K, Holm SE, Grahn Håkansson E, Nowrouzian F, Ivarsson M, Adlerberth I, Wold AE. Spray bacteriotherapy decreases middle ear fluid in children with secretory otitis media. *Arch Dis Child.* 2009 Feb;94(2):92-8.

Solomons NW, Guerrero AM, Torun B. Effective in vivo hydrolysis of milk lactose by beta-galactosidases in the presence of solid foods. *Am J Clin Nutr.* 1985 Feb;41(2):222-7.

Stadlbauer V, Mookerjee RP, Hodges S, Wright GA, Davies NA, Jalan R. Effect of probiotic treatment on deranged neutrophil function and cytokine responses in patients with compensated alcoholic cirrhosis. *J Hepatol.* 2008 Jun;48(6):945-51.

Stratiki Z, Costalos C, Sevastiadou S, Kastanidou O, Skouroliakou M, Giakoumatou A, Petrohilou V. The effect of a bifidobacter supplemented bovine milk on intestinal permeability of preterm infants. *Early Hum Dev.* 2007 Sep;83(9):575-9.

Strozzi GP, Mogna L. Quantification of folic acid in human feces after administration of *Bifidobacterium* probiotic strains. *J Clin Gastroenterol.* 2008 Sep;42 Suppl 3 Pt 2:S179-84.

Sturtzel B, Mikulits C, Gisinger C, Elmadfa I. Use of fiber instead of laxative treatment in a geriatric hospital to improve the wellbeing of seniors. *J Nutr Health Aging.* 2009 Feb;13(2):136-9.

Su P, Henriksson A, Tandianus JE, Park JH, Foong F, Dunn NW. Detection and quantification of *Bifidobacterium lactis* LAFTI B94 in human faecal samples from a consumption trial. *FEMS Microbiol Lett.* 2005 Mar 1;244(1):99-103.

Sugawara G, Nagino M, Nishio H, Ebata T, Takagi K, Asahara T, Nomoto K, Nimura Y. Perioperative synbiotic treatment to prevent postoperative infectious complications in biliary cancer surgery: a randomized controlled trial. *Ann Surg.* 2006 Nov;244(5):706-14.

Sullivan A, Barkholt L, Nord CE. *Lactobacillus acidophilus, Bifidobacterium lactis* and *Lactobacillus* F19 prevent antibiotic-associated ecological disturbances of Bacteroides fragilis in the intestine. *J Antimicrob Chemother.* 2003 Aug;52(2):308-11.

Szymański H, Chmielarczyk A, Strus M, Pejcz J, Jawień M, Kochan P, Heczko PB. Colonisation of the gastrointestinal tract by probiotic *L. rhamnosus* strains in acute diarrhoea in children. *Dig Liver Dis.* 2006 Dec;38 Suppl 2:S274-6.

Szymański H, Pejcz J, Jawień M, Chmielarczyk A, Strus M, Heczko PB. Treatment of acute infectious diarrhoea in infants and children with a mixture of three *Lactobacillus rhamnosus* strains—a randomized, double-blind, placebo-controlled trial. *Aliment Pharmacol Ther.* 2006 Jan 15;23(2):247-53.

Takagi A, Ikemura H, Matsuzaki T, Sato M, Nomoto K, Morotomi M, Yokokura T. Relationship between the in vitro response of dendritic cells to *Lactobacillus* and prevention of tumorigenesis in the mouse. *J Gastroenterol.* 2008;43(9):661-9.

Takeda K, Okumura K. Effects of a fermented milk drink containing *Lactobacillus casei* strain Shirota on the human NK-cell activity. *J Nutr.* 2007 Mar;137(3 Suppl 2):791S-3S.

Takeda K, Suzuki T, Shimada SI, Shida K, Nanno M, Okumura K. Interleukin-12 is involved in the enhancement of human natural killer cell activity by *Lactobacillus casei* Shirota. *Clin Exp Immunol.* 2006 Oct;146(1):109-15.

Tamura M, Shikina T, Morihana T, Hayama M, Kajimoto O, Sakamoto A, Kajimoto Y, Watanabe O, Nonaka C, Shida K, Nanno M. Effects of probiotics on allergic rhinitis induced by Japanese cedar pollen: randomized double-blind, placebo-controlled clinical trial. *Int Arch Allergy Imml.* 2007;143(1):75-82.

Tasli L, Mat C, De Simone C, Yazici H. Lactobacilli lozenges in the management of oral ulcers of Behçet's syndrome. *Clin Exp Rheumatol.* 2006 Sep-Oct;24(5 Suppl 42):S83-6.

Teitelbaum J. *From Fatigue to Fantastic.* New York: Avery, 2001.

Tevini M, ed. *UV-B Radiation and Ozone Depletion: Effects on humans, animals, plants, microorganisms and materials.* Boca Raton: Lewis Pub, 1993.

Thibault H, Aubert-Jacquin C, Goulet O. Effects of long-term consumption of a fermented infant formula (with *Bifidobacterium breve* c50 and *Streptococcus thermophilus* 065) on acute diarrhea in healthy infants. *J Pediatr Gastroenterol Nutr.* 2004 Aug;39(2):147-52.

Thomas Y, Schiff M, Belkadi L, Jurgens P, Kahhak L, Benveniste J. Activation of human neutrophils by electronically transmitted phorbol-myristate acetate. *Med Hypoth.* 2000;54: 33-39.

Thompson D. *On Growth and Form.* Cambridge: Cambridge University Press, 1992.

Tietze H. *Kombucha: The Miracle Fungus.* Gateway Books: Bath, UK, 1995.

Tormo Carnicer R, Infante Piña D, Roselló Mayans E, Bartolomé Comas R. Intake of fermented milk containing *Lactobacillus casei* DN-114 001 and its effect on gut flora. *An Pediatr.* 2006 Nov;65(5):448-53.

REFERENCES AND BIBLIOGRAPHY

Touhami M, Boudraa G, Mary JY, Soltana R, Desjeux JF. Clinical consequences of replacing milk with yogurt in persistent infantile diarrhea. *Ann Pediatr.* 1992 Feb;39(2):79-86.

Trenev N. *Probiotics: Nature's Internal Healers.* New York: Avery, 1998.

Trois L, Cardoso EM, Miura E. Use of probiotics in HIV-infected children: a randomized double-blind controlled study. *J Trop Pediatr.* 2008 Feb;54(1):19-24.

Tsuchiya J, Barreto R, Okura R, Kawakita S, Fesce E, Marotta F. Single-blind follow-up study on the effectiveness of a symbiotic preparation in irritable bowel syndrome. *Chin J Dig Dis.* 2004;5(4):169-74.

Tubelius P, Stan V, Zachrisson A. Increasing work-place healthiness with the probiotic *Lactobacillus reuteri*: a randomised, double-blind placebo-controlled study. *Environ Health.* 2005 Nov 7;4:25.

Tuomilehto J, Lindström J, Hyyrynen J, Korpela R, Karhunen ML, Mikkola L, Jauhiainen T, Seppo L, Nissinen A. Effect of ingesting sour milk fermented using *Lactobacillus helveticus* bacteria producing tripeptides on blood pressure in subjects with mild hypertension. *J Hum Hypertens.* 2004 Nov;18(11):795-802.

Turchet P, Laurenzano M, Auboiron S, Antoine JM. Effect of fermented milk containing the probiotic *Lactobacillus casei* DN-114001 on winter infections in free-living elderly subjects: a randomised, controlled pilot study. *J Nutr Health Aging.* 2003;7(2):75-7.

Tursi A, Brandimarte G, Giorgetti GM, Elisei W. Mesalazine and/or *Lactobacillus casei* in maintaining long-term remission of symptomatic uncomplicated diverticular disease of the colon. *Hepatogastroenterology.* 2008 May-Jun;55(84):916-20.

Twetman S, Derawi B, Keller M, Ekstrand K, Yucel-Lindberg T, Stecksen-Blicks C. Short-term effect of chewing gums containing probiotic *Lactobacillus reuteri* on the levels of inflammatory mediators in gingival crevicular fluid. *Acta Odontol Scand.* 2009 Feb;67(1):19-24.

Unknown. Proteolytic activity of various lactic acid bacteria. *Japan Jnl Dairy Food Sci.* 1990;39(4).

Vakil JR, Shahani KM. Carbohydrate metabolism of lactic acid cultures. V. Lactobionate and gluconate metabolism of *Streptococcus lactis* UN. *J Dairy Sci.* 1969 Dec;52(12):1928-34.

Valeur N, Engel P, Carbajal N, Connolly E, Ladefoged K. Colonization and immunomodulation by *Lactobacillus reuteri* ATCC 55730 in the human gastrointestinal tract. *Appl Environ Microbiol.* 2004 Feb;70(2):1176-81.

van Baarlen P, Troost FJ, van Hemert S, van der Meer C, de Vos WM, de Groot PJ, Hooiveld GJ, Brummer RJ, Kleerebezem M. Differential NF-kappaB pathways induction by *Lactobacillus plantarum* in the duodenum of healthy humans correlating with immune tolerance. *Proc Natl Acad Sci U S A.* 2009 Feb 17;106(7):2371-6

van den Heuvel EG, Schoterman MH, Muijs T. Transgalactooligosaccharides stimulate calcium absorption in postmenopausal women. *J Nutr.* 2000 Dec;130(12):2938-42.

Vendt N, Grünberg H, Tuure T, Malminiemi O, Wuolijoki E, Tillmann V, Sepp E, Korpela R. Growth during the first 6 months of life in infants using formula enriched with *Lactobacillus rhamnosus* GG: double-blind, randomized trial. *J Hum Nutr Diet.* 2006 Feb;19(1):51-8.

Venturi A, Gionchetti P, Rizzello F, Johansson R, Zucconi E, Brigidi P, Matteuzzi D, Campieri M. Impact on the composition of the faecal flora by a new probiotic preparation: preliminary data on maintenance treatment of patients with ulcerative colitis. *Aliment Pharmacol Ther.* 1999 Aug;13(8):1103-8.

Villarruel G, Rubio DM, Lopez F, Cintioni J, Gurevech R, Romero G, Vandenplas Y. *Saccharomyces boulardii* in acute childhood diarrhoea: a randomized, placebo-controlled study. *Acta Paediatr.* 2007 Apr;96(4):538-41.

Vivatvakin B, Kowitdamrong E. Randomized control trial of live *Lactobacillus acidophilus* plus *Bifidobacterium infantis* in treatment of infantile acute watery diarrhea. *J Med Assoc Thai.* 2006 Sep;89 Suppl 3:S126-33.

Wang KY, Li SN, Liu CS, Perng DS, Su YC, Wu DC, Jan CM, Lai CH, Wang TN, Wang WM. Effects of ingesting *Lactobacillus*- and *Bifidobacterium*-containing yogurt in subjects with colonized *Helicobacter pylori*. *Am J Clin Nutr.* 2004 Sep;80(3):737-41.

Watson L. *Supernature.* New York: Bantam, 1973.

Watve MG, Tickoo R, Jog MM, Bhole BD. How many antibiotics are produced by the genus Streptomyces? *Arch Microbiol.* 2001 Nov;176(5):386-90.

Weizman Z, Asli G, Alsheikh A. Effect of a probiotic infant formula on infections in child care centers: comparison of two probiotic agents. *Pediatrics.* 2005 Jan;115(1):5-9.

Weekes DJ. Management of Herpes Simplex with Virostatic Bacterial Agent. *EENT Dig.* 1963;25(12).

Weekes DJ. The treatment of aphthous stomatitis with Lactobacillus tablets. *NY State J Med.* 1958 Aug 15;58(16):2672-3.

Wenus C, Goll R, Loken EB, Biong AS, Halvorsen DS, Florholmen J. Prevention of antibiotic-associated diarrhoea by a fermented probiotic milk drink. *Eur J Clin Nutr.* 2008 Feb;62(2):299-301.

West R. Risk of death in meat and non-meat eaters. *BMJ.* 1994 Oct 8;309(6959):955.

Wheeler JG, Bogle ML, Shema SJ, Shirrell MA, Stine KC, Pittler AJ, Burks AW, Helm RM. Impact of dietary yogurt on immune function. *Am J Med Sci.* 1997 Feb;313(2):120-3.

Wheeler JG, Shema SJ, Bogle ML, Shirrell MA, Burks AW, Pittler A, Helm RM. Immune and clinical impact of *Lactobacillus acidophilus* on asthma. *Ann Allergy Asthma Immunol.* 1997 Sep;79(3):229-33.

Whorwell PJ, Altringer L, Morel J, Bond Y, Charbonneau D, O'Mahony L, Kiely B, Shanahan F, Quigley EM. Efficacy of an encapsulated probiotic *Bifidobacterium infantis* 35624 in women with irritable bowel syndrome. *Am J Gastroenterol.* 2006 Jul;101(7):1581-90.

Wickens K, Black PN, Stanley TV, Mitchell E, Fitzharris P, Tannock GW, Purdie G, Crane J; Probiotic Study Group. A differential effect of 2 probiotics in the prevention of eczema and atopy: a double-blind, randomized, placebo-controlled trial. *J Allergy Clin Immunol.* 2008 Oct;122(4):788-94.

Wildt S, Munck LK, Vinter-Jensen L, Hanse BF, Nordgaard-Lassen I, Christensen S, Avnstroem S, Rasmussen SN, Rumessen JJ. Probiotic treatment of collagenous colitis: a randomized, double-blind, placebo-controlled trial with *Lactobacillus acidophilus* and *Bifidobacterium animalis* subsp. *Lactis. Inflamm Bowel Dis.* 2006 May;12(5):395-401.

Williams AB, Yu C, Tashima K, Burgess J, Danvers K. Evaluation of two self-care treatments for prevention of vaginal candidiasis in women with HIV. *J Assoc Nurses AIDS Care.* 2001 Jul-Aug;12(4):51-7.

Witsell DL, Garrett CG, Yarbrough WG, Dorrestein SP, Drake AF, Weissler MC. Effect of *Lactobacillus acidophilus* on antibiotic-associated gastrointestinal morbidity: a prospective randomized trial. *J Otolaryngol.* 1995 Aug;24(4):230-3.

Wu Q, Wu K, Ye Y, Dong X, Zhang J. Quorum sensing and its roles in pathogenesis among animal-associated pathogens--a review. *Wei Sheng Wu Xue Bao.* 2009 Jul 4;49(7):853-8.

Xiao JZ, Kondo S, Takahashi N, Miyaji K, Oshida K, Hiramatsu A, Iwatsuki K, Kokubo S, Hosono A. Effects of milk products fermented by *Bifidobacterium longum* on blood lipids in rats and healthy adult male volunteers. *J Dairy Sci.* 2003 Jul;86(7):2452-61.

Xiao JZ, Kondo S, Yanagisawa N, Miyaji K, Enomoto K, Sakoda T, Iwatsuki K, Enomoto T. Clinical efficacy of probiotic *Bifidobacterium longum* for the treatment of symptoms of Japanese cedar pollen allergy in subjects evaluated in an environmental exposure unit. *Allergol Int.* 2007 Mar;56(1):67-75.

Xiao JZ, Kondo S, Yanagisawa N, Takahashi N, Odamaki T, Iwabuchi N, Miyaji K, Iwatsuki K, Togashi H, Enomoto K, Enomoto T. Probiotics in the treatment of Japanese cedar pollinosis: a double-blind placebo-controlled trial. *Clin Exp Allergy.* 2006 Nov;36(11):1425-35.

Xiao JZ, Kondo S, Yanagisawa N, Takahashi N, Odamaki T, Iwabuchi N, Iwatsuki K, Kokubo S, Togashi H, Enomoto K, Enomoto T. Effect of probiotic *Bifidobacterium longum* BB536 in relieving clinical symptoms and modulating plasma cytokine levels of Japanese cedar pollinosis during the pollen season. A randomized double-blind, placebo-controlled trial. *J Investig Allergol Clin Immunol.* 2006;16(2):86-93.

Xiao SD, Zhang DZ, Lu H, Jiang SH, Liu HY, Wang GS, Xu GM, Zhang ZB, Lin GJ, Wang GL. Multicenter, randomized, controlled trial of heat-killed *Lactobacillus acidophilus* LB in patients with chronic diarrhea. *Adv Ther.* 2003 Sep-Oct;20(5):253-60.

Yadav H, Jain S, Sinha PR. Antidiabetic effect of probiotic dahl containing *Lactobacillus acidophilus* and *Lactobacillus casei* in high fructose fed rats. *Nutrition.* 2007 Jan;23(1):62-8.

Yamamura S, Morishima H, Kumano-go T, Suganuma N, Matsumoto H, Adachi H, Sigedo Y, Mikami A, Kai T, Masuyama A, Takano T, Sugita Y, Takeda M. The effect of *Lactobacillus helveticus* fermented milk on sleep and health perception in elderly subjects. *Eur J Clin Nutr.* 2009 Jan;63(1):100-5.

Yasuda T, Takeyama Y, Ueda T, Shinzeki M, Sawa H, Nakajima T, Kuroda Y. Breakdown of Intestinal Mucosa Via Accelerated Apoptosis Increases Intestinal Permeability in Experimental Severe Acute Pancreatitis. *J Surg Res.* 2006 Apr 4.

Yeager S. The Doctor's Book of Food Remedies. Emmaus, PA: Rodale Press, 1998.

Zarate G, Gonzalez S, Chaia AP. *Assessing survival of dairy propionibacteria in gastrointestinal conditions and adherence to intestinal epithelia.* Centro de Referencia para Lactobacilos-CONICET. Tucuman, Argentina: Humana Press. 2004.

Zeng J, Li YQ, Zuo XL, Zhen YB, Yang J, Liu CH. Clinical trial: effect of active lactic acid bacteria on mucosal barrier function in patients with diarrhoea-predominant irritable bowel syndrome. *Aliment Pharmacol Ther.* 2008 Oct 15;28(8):994-1002.

Zhao HY, Wang HJ, Lu Z, Xu SZ. Intestinal microflora in patients with liver cirrhosis. *Chin J Dig Dis.* 2004;5(2):64-7.

Ziemniak W. Efficacy of *Helicobacter pylori* eradication taking into account its resistance to antibiotics. *J Physiol Pharmacol.* 2006 Sep;57 Suppl 3:123-41.

Zwolińska-Wcisło M, Brzozowski T, Mach T, Budak A, Trojanowska D, Konturek PC, Pajdo R, Drozdowicz D, Kwiecień S. Are probiotics effective in the treatment of fungal colonization of the gastrointestinal tract? Experimental and clinical studies. *J Physiol Pharmacol.* 2006 Nov;57 Suppl 9:35-49.

Index

Breinigsville, PA USA
07 May 2010
237579BV00001B/22/P